PSYCHOSOCIAL ASPECTS OF CANCER PATIENT CARE

A Self-Instructional Text

PSYCHOSOCIAL ASPECTS OF CANCER PATIENT CARE

A Self-Instructional Text

Elizabeth A. Smith, Ph.D.

Assistant Professor of Psychology
The University of Texas Health Science Center at Houston
Division of Continuing Education
Consultant to the Office of Education
The University of Texas System Cancer Center
M. D. Anderson Hospital and Tumor Institute, Houston

McGraw-Hill Book Company

A Blakiston Publication

New York   St. Louis   San Francisco   Auckland   Düsseldorf   Johannesburg
Kuala Lumpur   London   Mexico   Montreal   New Delhi   Panama
Paris   São Paulo   Singapore   Sydney   Tokyo   Toronto

Notice

Medicine is an ever-changing science. As new research and clinical experience broaden our knowledge, changes in treatment and drug therapy are required. The editors and the publisher of this work have made every effort to ensure that the drug dosage schedules herein are accurate and in accord with the standards accepted at the time of publication. Readers are advised, however, to check the product information sheet included in the package of each drug they plan to administer to be certain that changes have not been made in the recommended dose or in the contraindications for administration. This recommendation is of particular importance in regard to new or infrequently used drugs.

Companion text by Elizabeth A. Smith, **A Comprehensive Approach to Rehabilitation of the Cancer Patient.** This project was supported by Texas Regional Medical Program, Inc., Contract Number 75-111G and The University of Texas Health Science Center at Houston, Division of Continuing Education.

Library of Congress Cataloging in Publication Data

Smith, Elizabeth A   date
    Psychosocial aspects of cancer patient care.

    "A Blakiston publication."
    Contract no. 75-111G.
    1. Cancer nursing. 2. Cancer patients—Rehabilitation. 3. Cancer—Psychological aspects. I. Title. [DNLM: 1. Neoplasms—Nursing—Programmed texts. 2. Nurse-patient relations—Programmed texts. 3. Terminal care—Programmed texts. WY18 S646p 1975a]
RC266.S63   610.73′6   76-2059
ISBN 0-07-058493-1

CONTENTS

PREFACE

The material selected for inclusion in this self-instructional text represents a small sample of the volumes of information available on cancer. Although psychosocial literature is extensive, it has not been incorporated into any unified whole. Our concerted effort has been, therefore, to reinterpret commonly accepted psychological concepts and methods within the context of cancer patient care.

The self-instructional text is designed for the health care professional whose knowledge of cancer and of basic psychological terms, concepts, and methods used in cancer patient care is limited; among these persons are nurses, occupational therapists, physical therapists, speech therapists, enterostomal therapists, vocational counselors, social workers, clinical psychologists, chaplains, and other members of the health care team. Experienced health care professionals may also use this text for review or for teaching purposes.

Since the major focus of the text is on psychosocial aspects related to care of the cancer patient, many medical elements had to be omitted, and those that were of necessity included had to be treated in the broadest of terms.

All materials for this text and for the companion text, *A Comprehensive Approach to the Rehabilitation of the Cancer Patient,* were developed with Regional Medical Program of Texas contract funds awarded for the period August 15, 1974 to June 24, 1975. This 10-month period was entirely too short to adequately develop, test out, and revise all materials. Your assistance in this testing and revising process will provide meaningful information which hopefully can be incorporated into a second edition. Please send your questions, corrections, and suggestions to me at the following address:

Elizabeth A. Smith, Ph.D.
The University of Texas Health Science Center at Houston
Division of Continuing Education
Office of Health Education
Houston, Texas 77025

Acknowledgments

I wish to acknowledge the assistance of the health care professionals who so generously devoted their time to serve as consultants and reviewers. Their constructive comments and suggestions were greatly appreciated, and contributed to the overall quality of this self-instructional text. I am particularly indebted to Mrs. Grace Gilkeson, M.A., O.T.R., faculty member, Texas Woman's University, Houston; Mr. Jeffrey Kudsk, L.P.T., M.A., faculty member, University of Iowa, Iowa City, Iowa; and Wallace S. Tirman, M.D., South Bend, Indiana.

My experience as evaluator for ongoing National Cancer Institute funded training programs titled Oncology Nursing, Cancer Training: A Continuing Education Program for Physical and Occupational Therapists, and Training of Professional Teams in Cancer Rehabilitation, awarded to the University of Texas System Cancer Center, M. D. Anderson Hospital and Tumor Institute, provided basic information on both psychosocial aspects of cancer patient care and on rehabilitation.

My association with Miss Renilda Hilkemeyer, R.N., B.S., Director, Department of Nursing, M. D. Anderson Hospital, and with Miss Catherine Herrington, R.N., B.S., Mrs. Patricia Kuykendall, R.N., B.S., M.S.Nr., Mrs. Sue Walker, R.N., B.S., who performed chapter reviews, enabled me to develop a perspective in the broad areas of nursing and rehabilitation.

I wish to express my appreciation to the following persons from the University of Texas Health Science Center at Houston, Division of Continuing Education: Grant Taylor, M.D., Director, for his encouragement and support throughout the preparation of the text. I am deeply indebted to Miss Annie Morris, B.A., who so willingly and enthusiastically functioned as a research and editorial assistant. The patience and diligence she exhibited throughout the process of writing, revising, and typing was greatly appreciated. I also wish to acknowledge the assistance of Mr. Bobby Brown, Mrs. Patricia LaReau, B.A., Grayce Scarborough, Susan Warley, and other employees of the Division of Continuing Education who assisted in the varied activities directly associated with the preparation of this self-instructional text.

The contribution of the students who worked through the texts, evaluated the various chapters, and made suggestions for improvement were of great value.

Elizabeth A. Smith

INSTRUCTIONS TO THE READER

The narrative method of presentation used in this self-instructional text does not follow the traditional format, as material on cancer and on psychosocial aspects was considered too comprehensive to be presented in small, discrete units. Chapters have been divided into two or more sections, each of which is followed by a reinforcement and review section designed to test acquisition of knowledge. You will be required to:

1. Master certain basic cancer facts, which include methods used in detection, treatment, and control.
2. Recall definitions for commonly used psychosocial and medical terms and incorporate them into your working vocabulary.
3. Demonstrate understanding of frequently used psychological concepts and methods and their relevance to patient care.
4. Apply newly acquired knowledge to the development of skills related to (a) observing, (b) evaluating, (c) reacting to, and (d) predicting the most frequently occurring behavior of cancer patients.

Suggestions for Use

In order to derive maximum benefit from this self-instructional text, the following sequence of steps is recommended:

1. If you wish to use the *same test* for pre- and post-testing purposes, respond to all questions both *before* and *after* working through the chapters. Two answer sheets have been provided. If you do not want to take the *same* pre- and post-test, respond to the even-numbered questions for the pre-test and the odd-numbered questions for the post-test, or conversely. It is also possible to use each chapter test for pre- and post-testing purposes. The minimum standards you or your instructor may set for performance are an individual matter. The important factor is that you satisfactorily demonstrate to yourself that knowledge has been acquired. Applying this knowledge is an even greater challenge.
2. Read each section of each chapter with the goal of understanding in mind. Since the material is both comprehensive and condensed, you may have to reread and carefully study certain sections. You may wish to underline key words or phrases or write notes in the margins. Definitions presented at the end of each chapter and reference materials in the Appendix may need to be consulted. In some instances, you may wish to look up references or refer to materials listed in the suggested readings sections.
3. Answer each question in the reinforcement and review sections. If you have difficulty in writing out complete answers, you may need to reread information presented in the immediately preceding section. Only after you have made a concerted effort to provide complete answers to *all* questions should you consult the an-

swer section. If your answers are incomplete or inaccurate, you should write out a complete answer as this effort is reinforcing.

The estimated time to complete each chapter ranges from 40 minutes for short chapters to over 2 hours for long chapters.

Ideally, persons working through self-instructional materials should have personal contact with an instructor or resource person. Since this personal form of contact is seldom possible, an effort was made to anticipate problem areas and to provide detailed answers to most of the questions in the reinforcement and review sections. The levels of response required in the reinforcement and review sections range from simple recall of facts to creative application of knowledge in a patient care setting. It is hoped that the reader will be stimulated by this approach.

Since feedback is such a valuable component of any learning process, it would be greatly appreciated if you would complete the evaluation on page 181 of this self-instructional text and mail it to the address given at the conclusion of the Preface.

Elizabeth A. Smith

Chapter 1

WHAT IS CANCER?

Historical Beginnings

"Cancer in the ancestral species of man is more than a million years old."[13(p83)] The earliest written records of man contain descriptions of abnormalities of the uterus, skin, bones, and breasts. Evidence of cancer has been found in skeletons of prehistoric animals and in Etruscan, Peruvian, and Egyptian mummies.[6,13]

Descriptions of cancer symptoms and treatment methods, such as the use of a knife, date back to 2500 B.C. Hippocrates' writings include descriptions of cancer of the breast, uterus, stomach, skin, and rectum. "Black bile" was mainly responsible for cancer according to Hippocrates. The term "carcinoma" stems from the Greek word karkinos (crab) and was inherited from Hippocrates.

The first cancer surgery was performed by Cornelius Celsus, a Roman physician, in the first century A.D. In the second and third centuries A.D., surgical techniques, such as those used in mastectomies, were improved. During these years, the pain and suffering caused by cancer was alleviated by poppy seed infusions.[13]

In the Middle Ages, discoveries made by Arabian, French, and German surgeons greatly contributed to the steadily increasing fund of knowledge about cancer. Advances made in the last 20 years in pathology, surgery, epidemiology, and treatment methods, to mention only a few areas, are too numerous to be included. Additional information may be obtained from the sources cited in the "Suggested Readings" section at the end of this chapter.

Definition

No single definition of cancer is universally acceptable. Some of the many definitions of cancer include[13,17]:

1. cellular tissue in which the normal growth and division controlling mechanisms have been permanently impaired permitting progressive growth or spreading through the blood stream or lymph system.

2. a genetic disease of somatic cells caused by a mutation of a previously normal cell into a new and malignant cell.

3. a spontaneous autoagressive disease of a tissue initiated by random gene mutation in a stem cell.

4. a group of diseases of unknown and possibly multiple causes, occurring in all human and animal populations, and arising in all tissues composed of potentially dividing cells.

Cancer cells may also form masses which impede the function of the tissue. The symptoms, course, treatment, and prognosis are related specifically to the organ invaded and its normal function.[4]

Cancers (1) differ in tissues of origin and structural appearance, (2) arise from different causes, (3) have varying clinical courses, and (4) appear in individuals of divergent sex, age, and physiological and psychological characteristics.[4]

The term "oncology" is frequently used in connection with cancer. Oncology is the study of a large variety of tumors or swellings. Tumors are classified as benign and malignant. The benign tumor does not usually invade the normal tissue around it. The malignant tumor invades the surrounding tissue and also gives rise to metastases (secondary growths) in other parts of the body.[1] Malignant tumors may cause death.[14]

Classifications

Although there are approximately 300 different types of cancers,[16] the two main classifications are: (1) carcinomas, which invade the skin and lining of hollow organs and passageways and (2) sarcomas, which attack bone, muscle, cartilage, and the lymph system.[10]

Cause of Cancer

The exact cause of cancer is unknown. Although there are readily recognizable histo-pathologic differences between the cancer cell and the normal cell, few metabolic differences have been determined. With increasing knowledge of DNA, a common ground for carcinogenesis of hereditary, viral, chemical, and radiation factors has been postulated.[14] Epidemiologic studies which seek to discover the vectors or agents in disease have revealed many new clues regarding the origin of cancer.

Spratt[16] states that there have been over 30 recent reports indicating a relationship between various forms of cancer and diet. In most instances, organs of the digestive tract have been involved, but diet has been associated with cancer of the bladder, liver, and prostate. Spratt offers practical suggestions regarding diets associated with low incidences of various forms of cancer.

The following conditions are often connected with abnormal cell growth and may be cited as possible causative factors[10]:

1. mechanical--Examples include chronic irritation of warts or moles, excessive rubbing of mouth tissue from pipestems, badly fitting dentures, etc.

2. chemical--Examples include carcinogenic substances such as coal tars, irritants in cigarette smoke, arsenical compounds, some dyes, etc.

3. radiation--Examples include prolonged overexposure to the sun's ultraviolet (tanning) rays or overexposure to X-ray, radium, radioactive isotopes, etc.

4. viral--A virus is an ultramicroscopic infectious agent that reproduces only in living cells. The viral theory is controversial.

Although cancers may arise following any of the stimuli listed above, there is usually a prolonged latent period before any abnormal cell reproduction begins.[17]

In some instances, precancerous conditions such as leukoplasia and and keratosis may develop into cancer.

Spread

The main ways in which cancer spreads are: (1) local extension or infiltration. As cancer cells multiply, they invade surrounding tissue and continue to grow; (2) metastasis. Cancer cells are carried by blood or the lymph system from primary tumors to other parts of the body such as the lung and brain where they form new growths.[10]

Reinforcement and Review

1.1 Which of the following statements are true? Circle the correct
response(s).

   1. The first descriptions of cancer surgery date back
       to 2500 B.C.
   2. The term "carcinoma," meaning cancer, is of recent
       origin.
   3. There was no anesthetic for the cancer surgery per-
       formed in the Middle Ages.
   4. Mastectomies have been performed for 1,700 to 1,800
       years.
   5. The first cancer surgery was performed in the first
       century A.D.
   6. Evidence of cancer has been detected in the skeletons
       of prehistoric animals and in Egyptian, Peruvian, and
       Etruscan mummies.

1.2 Which of the following phrases most closely describe cancer?

   1. a recently discovered disease.
   2. normal biologic process.
   3. a disease which occurs only in humans.
   4. spreads through the blood stream or lymph system.
   5. uncontrolled multiplication of cells.
   6. does not impede the function of the tissue, bone, or muscle.
   7. the study of malignant tumors.
   8. may be caused by mutation of a previously normal
       cell into a new and malignant cell.

1.3 The two main classifications of cancer are:

       _____ and _____ .

1.4 Cancer which invades the skin and lining of hollow organs and passageways is:

       _____

1.5 Sarcomas attack:

       _____ , _____ , and _____ .

1.6 Emotional status of the patient affects the course of the disease.

       ___true/___false

1.7 Cancer spreads by:

_____ and _____.

1.8 The four main postulated causes of cancer are:

_____, _____, _____, and _____.

1.9 Identify by writing "mechanical," "chemical," "radiation," or "viral" which of the listed conditions may be connected with abnormal cell growth.

   1. irritants in cigarette smoke _____
   2. chronic irritation of warts or moles_____
   3. certain dyes_____
   4. prolonged exposure to sun's ultraviolet rays_____
   5. excessive rubbing of mouth tissue from pipestems_____

Answers to Questions 1.1 - 1.9

1.1 1, 4, 5, and 6.

1.2 4, 5, and 8.

1.3 carcinomas, sarcomas.

1.4 carcinomas.

1.5 bone, muscle, cartilage, and lymph system.

1.6 true.

1.7 local extension (infiltration) and metastasis.

1.8 can not be specified, but there is a common ground in hereditary, viral,
     chemical, and radiation factors.

1.9 (1) chemical. (2) mechanical. (3) chemical. (4) radiation. (5)
     mechanical.

Cancer Incidence

The incidence of cancer is rising about 2% each year. Cancer affects every age group, both sexes, and every part of the body.[1] The following statistics are from the American Cancer Society[2]:

1. About 53,000,000 Americans now living will eventually have cancer.

2. In the 1970s, there will be an estimated 6,500,000 new cancer cases, and more than 10,000,000 under medical care for cancer.

3. In 1975, there will be about 665,000 new cases of cancer. This figure does not include superficial skin cancer or carcinoma-in-situ of the uterine cervix.

4. In 1975, more than 1,000,000 Americans will receive medical care for cancer.

5. There are now 1,500,000 Americans alive today who have been "cured" of cancer. "Cured" means that they are without evidence of the disease at least five years after diagnosis and treatment. The decision as to when a patient may be considered cured is made by the individual physician. While some patients may be discharged as cancer free after one year, others may be similarly discharged after three or after five years.

Based on statistics presented in the following table, "Cancer Incidence by Site and Sex," the three most common major sites of cancer for men are: (1) lung--22%, (2) prostate--17%, and (3) colon and rectum--14%. Corresponding percentages for women are: (1) breast--27%, (2) colon and rectum--15%, and (3) uterus--14%.

CANCER INCIDENCE BY SITE AND SEX[2]

(Excluding superficial skin cancer
and carcinoma-in-situ of uterine cervix)

Male	Female
skin.........................1%	skin.........................1%
oral.........................5%	oral.........................2%
lung........................22%	breast......................27%
colon and rectum...........14%	lung.........................6%
other digestive............12%	colon and rectum...........15%
prostate....................17%	other digestive.............9%
urinary......................9%	uterus......................14%
leukemia and lymphomas.......8%	urinary......................4%
all other..................12%	leukemia and lymphomas.......7%
	all other..................15%

Cancer Deaths

More men than women die of cancer, with more than half of all deaths occurring after age 65.[1] The following statistics are from the American Cancer Society[2]:

1. Next to heart disease, cancer is America's leading cause of death, with over 365,000 deaths per year. In America, one out of every six deaths from all causes is from cancer.

2. In the 1970s, there will be an estimated 3,500,000 cancer deaths.

The two most significant trends in the age-adjusted cancer death rate are[2]:

1. a steady decline for women since 1936, with a total drop of 13%. This decrease in mortality is primarily attributable to a sharp reduction in mortality from cancer of the uterine cervix, a readily detectable disease.

2. a steady increase for men of 40% since 1930. This increase in mortality is primarily attributable to a 2,000% increase for lung cancer, a highly preventable disease.

Cancer is the leading cause of death from disease among children from one to fourteen years of age.[12] Each year approximately 3,500 children under the age of 15 die of cancer.[1] The two main types of cancer found in children are: leukemia and lymphoma(42%) and solid tumors (58%). The most common cancer sites in children are: bone marrow (leukemia), the brain or central nervous system (cerebellar astrocytoma), the lymph system (Hodgkin's disease), kidneys (Wilms' tumor), adrenals (neuroblastoma), bones (osteogenic sarcoma), and soft tissues (rhabdomyosarcoma).[12]

Statistics presented in the following table, "Cancer Deaths by Site and Sex," reveal that lung cancer accounts for 33% of cancer deaths in males and cancer of the breast accounts for 20% of cancer deaths in females.

CANCER DEATHS BY SITE AND SEX[2]

Male	Female
skin.........................1%	skin.........................1%
oral.........................3%	oral.........................1%
lung.........................33%	breast.......................20%
colon and rectum............12%	lung.........................11%
other digestive.............15%	colon and rectum............15%
prostate.....................9%	other digestive.............14%
urinary......................6%	uterus.......................7%
leukemia and lymphomas.......9%	urinary......................3%
all other...................12%	leukemia and lymphomas.......9%
	all other...................19%

Reinforcement and Review

1.10 The incidence of cancer is rising about _____% each year.

    1. 0.2%
    2. 0.5%
    3. 1.1%
    4. 2.0%
    5. 4.0%

1.11 In the 1970s, how many Americans will be under medical care for cancer?

    1.   1,000,000
    2.   5,000,000
    3. 10,000,000
    4. 16,000,000
    5. 23,000,000

1.12 Approximately how many Americans now living will eventually have cancer?

    1. 10,000,000
    2. 30,000,000
    3. 50,000,000
    4. 70,000,000
    5. 90,000,000

1.13 Cancer ranks _____ as America's leading cause of death.

    1. 1st
    2. 2nd
    3. 3rd
    4. 4th
    5. 5th

1.14 Approximately what percentage of deaths in America are caused by cancer?

    1. 25%
    2. 10%
    3.   6%
    4. 17%
    5. 33%

1.15 How many cancer deaths will there be in the 1970s?

      1. 3,500,000
      2. 6,500,000
      3. 7,500,000
      4. 8,000,000
      5. 8,500,000

1.16 Exclusive of superficial skin cancer and carcinoma-in-situ of the uterine cervix, how many new cases of cancer will there be in 1975?

      1. 150,000
      2. 350,000
      3. 475,000
      4. 500,000
      5. 665,000

1.17 How many Americans are currently receiving medical care for cancer?

      1.   500,000
      2.   750,000
      3. 1,000,000
      4. 1,500,000
      5. 2,000,000

1.18 How many Americans are presently without evidence of cancer five years following diagnosis and treatment?

      1. 1,000,000
      2. 1,500,000
      3. 2,000,000
      4. 2,500,000
      5. 3,000,000

1.19 For men, the most common major site of cancer is:

      1. colon and rectum
      2. prostate
      3. digestive tract
      4. skin
      5. lung

1.20 For women, the most common major site of cancer is:

      1. uterus
      2. breast

3. colon and rectum
4. urinary
5. lung

1.21 For children, the leading cause of death from disease is:

1. accidents
2. influenza
3. cancer
4. heart disease
5. certain diseases of early infancy

1.22 Each year approximately how many children under the age of 15 die from cancer?

1. 3,500
2. 4,000
3. 4,500
4. 5,000
5. 5,500

1.23 Since 1930, the age-adjusted rates for men reveal a ___% increase, which is primarily attributable to cancer of the _____.

1.24 Since 1936, the age-adjusted cancer rates for women reveal a ____% decrease, which is primarily attributable to detection of the_____.

Answers to Questions 1.10 - 1.24

1.10   (4) 2.0%

1.11   (3) 10,000,000

1.12   (3) 50,000,000

1.13   (2) 2nd

1.14   (4) 1 out of 6 or approximately 17%

1.15   (1) 3,500,000

1.16   (5) 665,000

1.17   (3) 1,000,000 (figures are projected for 1975)

1.18   (2) 1,500,000

1.19   (5) lung.

1.20   (2) breast.

1.21   (3) cancer.

1.22   (1) 3,500

1.23   40%, lung.

1.24   13%, cervix.

Possible Causes of Cancer

Facts and fiction about the cause of cancer[10]:

1. There is no proof that cancer is inherited--with the exception of
   Retinoblastoma, a rare type of eye cancer that is highly curable
   in early stages. Tendencies to develop cancer or environmental
   conditions and occupations that eventually result in cancer may
   run in families. Persons with chromosomal abnormalities such as
   those that occur in Mongolism or Down's syndrome illustrate the
   role of heredity in the development of cancer; these persons develop
   malignancies about ten times more often than would occur by chance.

2. Cancer is not contagious.

3. Experts generally agree that cigarette smoking is closely related to
   cancer. Heavy smokers have a 10 to 20 times higher incidence of
   lung cancer as nonsmokers.

4. A relationship between air pollution and cancer has been postulated
   but not confirmed. City air, however, contains as much as 16 times
   as many cancer-causing chemicals as noncity air.

5. There is no evidence that a single or occasional injury such as
   bruises or fractures can cause cancer.

6. There is no evidence that any food in the normal American diet
   definitely causes cancer--or that special diets can cure cancer.

Early Warning Signs

Early warning signs are extremely important. The following list is
published by the American Cancer Society[2]:

1. change in bowel or bladder habits.

2. a sore that does not heal.

3. unusual bleeding or discharge.

4. thickening or lump in breast or elsewhere.

5. indigestion or difficulty in swallowing.

6. obvious changes in wart or mole.

7. nagging cough or hoarseness.

If any of these warning signs is apparent, a thorough physical examination is warranted. The components of a good periodic examination have been presented by the American Cancer Society.[1]

Questionable signs require clinical testing and/or surgical intervention to establish or exclude the diagnosis.[14] Before tests and radiographic examinations are performed, an histologic diagnosis to determine the extent or stage and type of cancer is necessary.

An histological examination is a very important factor in establishing a definitive diagnosis and treatment. The groundwork, staging, classification, and other procedures must be either performed or discussed before the treatment plan is established. Radical treatment must not occur until the histologic diagnosis is made.

According to Rubin,[14] procedures used to define the exact extent of the disease include the following categories:

1. primary lesion--examination of accessible lesions and internal lesions such as cervix or bladder tumors (preferably under anesthesia). Radiographs of the site are made.

2. lymph nodes--Examinations of accessible nodes and inaccessible nodes (by needle biopsy) are performed. Lymphangiography may also be used.

3. metastases--examination of the lungs, liver, bone marrow, and

brain.   These areas are common sites for metastases.

Staging

A system of staging or classifying anatomic and histologic considerations is basic to understanding the nature and course of cancer. If any standardized nomenclature is to be developed, precise descriptive terms must be developed and utilized. Although there are many international committees* attempting to standardize nomenclature, the main problem is to keep the descriptions from being so complicated that they have little clinical usefulness.

According to the Commission on Clinical Oncology of the International Union Against Cancer, the objectives of staging are to:

1. aid the clinician in planning of treatment.

2. give some indication of prognosis.

3. assist in the evaluation of prognosis.

4. facilitate the exchange of information.

5. assist in the continuing investigation of cancer.

Survival

The five-year survival rate is commonly chosen as a parameter for measuring survival and for indicating the curability of the cancer. The computation of five-year survival rates must take into consideration the following factors:

1. accessibility of the cancer.

2. stage in which the cancer is detected.

---

* The Union Against Cancer and the American Joint Committee on Cancer Staging are two such committees.

3. effectiveness of treatment.

4. type of hosts harboring the cancer,

In general, assumptions regarding five-year survival are:

1. Females generally have better survival rates than males with the same cancer.

2. Many cancers are highly curable in localized stages. Curability is reduced by half or more when cancer is in a regionalized stage, i.e., has spread to regional lymph nodes.

3. The overall stage results, compared to the achievement in localized and regionalized stage results, tells how often the disease presents as a metastatic process.

4. Survival is generally better in cancers located in accessible sites than in cancers of internal origins. This finding indicates the importance of early detection.

Since each type of cancer has its specific prognosis, especially in the early clinically detectable stages, it is extremely difficult to present meaningful survival data. For example, 50% of all patients with the diagnosis of cancer of the lung are inoperable when first seen; approximately 25% of all patients survive 6 to 9 months, and only 2 1/2% of all patients survive for five years.[8] On the other hand, cancer of the cervix is highly treatable when initially detected (usually by a Pap smear), and complete cures are not uncommon. Most basic cancer texts provide comprehensive survival data. Publications by the American Cancer Society are an excellent source for current statistics.

In the early 1900s, few cancer patients had any hope of long-term survival. The survival rate has since increased from less than one-in-five in the 1930s to one-in-three in the 1970s. Of every six persons who get cancer today (exclusive of superficial skin cancer and carcinoma-in-situ of uterine cervix), two will be saved and four will die. Of these four who die, one might have been saved with early diagnosis and prompt treatment.[2]

Importance of Early Detection and Diagnosis

Early detection is the key to saving one-out-of-two persons who get cancer, rather than the present one-out-of-three. Although present treatment knowledge is adequate for this goal, timely detection and diagnosis lag behind.[2] In cancer more than in any other disease, an early diagnosis is significant. In many cases, such as cancer of the lung, cancer has reached advanced stages before the patient becomes aware of a difficulty that prompts him to seek medical advice.

Effective diagnosis is concerned with the identification of a specific type of cancer affecting a certain organ (site) or structure of a particular individual of a specific sex and age who has unique physiological and psychological characteristics. The extent of the malignancy and the presence or absence of metastasis must also be known. All of these factors are of extreme importance in the diagnosis and prognosis (medical prediction of the course and termination of the disease). Only with this information can definitive treatment take place.

Reinforcement and Review

1.25 1. Cancer is always inherited. ___true/___false

2. Heavy smokers have a 10 to 20 times higher incidence of lung cancer as nonsmokers. ___true/___false

3. Polluted air may contain cancer-causing chemicals. ___true/___false

4. Solitary bruises and fractures cause cancer. ___true/___false

5. Certain diets can help cure cancer. ___true/___false

6. There is a small positive correlation between the occurrence of Mongolism and leukemia. ___true/___false

1.26 List 5 early warning signs of cancer:

1. _____

2. _____

3. _____

4. _____

5. _____

1.27 The most important reasons for performing a complete histological examination are:

_____ and _____

1.28 What are the major reasons for developing a system of staging anatomic and histologic data?

1. _____

2. _____

3. _____

4. _____

5. _____

1.29 List the factors taken into consideration in the computation of five-year survival rates:

1. _____

2. _____

3. _____

4. _____

1.30 Current survival rates for cancer patients are:

1. 1 in 5
2. 1 in 4
3. 1 in 6
4. 1 in 3
5. 2 in 4

1.31 With early diagnosis and prompt treatment, survival rates could be increased to:

1. 1 in 3
2. 1 in 2
3. 1 in 4
4. 1 in 5
5. 1 in 6

1.32 Definitive treatment can not take place unless _____ and _____ are known.

Answers to Questions 1.25 - 1.32

1.25 (1) false. (2) true. (3) true. (4) false. (5) false. (6) true.

1.26 Any of the following are correct: (1) change in bowel, bladder habits.
(2) sore that does not heal. (3) unusual bleeding or discharge.
(4) thickening in breast or elsewhere. (5) indigestion, difficulty
in swallowing. (6) changes in wart or mole. (7) nagging cough.
Because of increased public awareness, early warning signs of breast
cancer are well known. However, few persons realize that warts, moles,
and sores that do not heal may be potentially cancerous.

1.27 (1) to determine the stage of cancer. (2) to determine the type of
cancer.

1.28 (1) aid in treatment planning. (2) simplify descriptions of cancer.
(3) aid in prognosis. (4) facilitate information exchange. (5) assist
in cancer research.

1.29 (1) accessibility of the cancer. (2) stage in which cancer is detected.
(3) effectiveness of treatment. (4) type of hosts harboring the cancer.

1.30 (4) 1 in 3.

1.31 (2) 1 in 2.

1.32 extent of the malignancy and presence or absence of metastasis.

Diagnostic Procedures

Some of the most common diagnostic procedures include:

1. bronchoscopy--examination of the bronchi through a tracheal wound or
   through a bronchoscope.

2. colonoscopy--use of a fibre-optic colonoscope which provides a view
   of the entire colon.

3. proctoscopy--inspection of the rectum with a proctoscope. (A sigmoidoscopy is probably a better procedure.)

4. sigmoidoscopy--inspection of the sigmoid flexure by the aid of a
   speculum (sigmoidoscope).

5. esophagoscopy--endoscopic examination of the esophagus.

6. lymphangiography--X-ray of the lymphatic vessels following injection
   of a contrast medium such as Ethiodol.

7. gastroscopy--the inspection of the interior of the stomach by means
   of the gastroscope.

8. arteriography--Arteriograms are obtained by injection of contrast
   media into the appropriate artery for the purposes of detecting
   tumors of the brain, kidney, liver, heart, and adrenal gland.[1]

9. X-ray--a photographic image produced by the action of X-rays or rays
   from radiographic substances.

10. nuclear medicine--a broad field of investigation which uses radio-
    isotopic techniques to determine the origin and extent of disease
    in various organ systems of the body.

11. thermography--a photographic representation of varying skin temper-
    atures of the breast. A heat-sensing device records localized skin
    temperatures and the elevations often found over inflammatory and

malignant lesions.

12. xeroradiography--an offshoot of mammography in which X-rays of the breast are made on xerographic plates instead of photographic film. In proper hands, this technique reveals more detail than a mammogram.

13. mammography--a soft tissue radiology technique useful in detecting and helping to diagnose cancer.

14. "Pap smear" (Papanicolaou's smear)--a method of collecting and staining cells developed by Dr. George Papanicolaou. Although this method is usually considered to be a means for detecting cervical cancer, it can also be used for collecting and staining any body secretions such as those from the lung and mouth.

Treatment of Cancer

Generally, treatment methods designed to kill cancer cells also kill normal cells. This method ensures that all, or the maximum number of cancer cells, are killed.

The treatment of cancer makes exceedingly heavy demands on the health care team.[11] Since the responsibility of treatment is great and judgment critical, only those capable professional persons who are properly trained should undertake treatment. Cobb[3] states that those responsible for developing the initial treatment plan include: (1) surgeon, (2) radiotherapist, (3) internist or family physician, (4) pathologist, (5) psychologist or psychiatrist, and (6) rehabilitation counselor.

The treatment plan must be flexible so that modifications may be made if surgical or pathological examinations so indicate.[4] These treatment plans must take into consideration the emotional and physical status of the patient. In planning for the emotional needs of the patient, a balance must exist between hope for a cure and reality. The "quality of survival" is a critical factor since the difference between merely being alive and leading a functional life is vast.

The extent of the treatment is determined by the following factors:

1. kind of cancer.

2. aggressiveness of the cancer.

3. predictability of the spread of cancer.

4. morbidity and mortality of the therapeutic procedure.

5. cure rate for the therapeutic procedure under consideration.

6. general health of the patient.

As the chance for cure decreases, the tendency to be more radical appears justified. However, the basic principle in treatment is to cure the patient with minimal physical and emotional impairments. A conservative approach may lead to recurrence, whereas a more radical approach may result in increased mortality. It is not always possible to strike a balance between conservative and radical approaches. This difficulty is attributed primarily to differences of opinion and patient-related variables rather than strictly to medical facts. Management problems and difficulties may result nevertheless.

Cancer is treated by: (1) surgery, (2) radiotherapy, (3) chemotherapy, (4) immunotherapy, (5) hormone therapy, or any combination of these methods. Other relatively new procedures may also be used. The use of each method and the order in which methods are used depends upon the various types, stages, and locations of the tumors. Methods are described below.

1. surgery--the most frequently used of the treatment methods. Surgery

is used to remove the tumor and a margin of surrounding normal
tissue. Cancer that has metastasized to lymph nodes requires an
"en bloc" resection of the primary site of malignant growth and the
lymph nodes of the area.[1] Examples of common cancers in which
surgery may be curative are: gastrointestinal (GI) cancers, bone,
breast, endometrium, eye, genitalia, in situ carcinoma of the cervix,
most skin cancers, and others.[1]

2. radiotherapy (Cobalt and Isotope) and X-ray therapy (XRT)--used
for cure or palliation in 50 to 60% of all cancer cases. Radiotherapy may be used before surgery to reduce the size of the tumor or
after surgery as a precaution against any existing scattered malignant cells. Radioactive substances may also be implanted in the
tumor.

3. chemotherapy--is used independently or in conjunction with surgery
and/or radiation therapy or XRT. Chemotherapy may be given to reduce
the size of the tumor. Types of chemicals used include: (1) alkylating agents, (2) antibiotic agents, (3) antimetabolites, and
(4) plant alkaloids. These chemicals, administered orally and intra-
venously, are most effective in retarding or preventing the DNA in the
cell from dividing. Chemotherapeutic agents have a deleterious effect
on the division of normal and abnormal cells. In certain types of
cancer and in advanced cases, chemotherapy may be used instead of
surgery. Chemotherapy was first used approximately 15 years ago.

4. immunotherapy--is used to stimulate host immunological competence
or to enhance the immunological response with active donor cells or
irradiated cultured host cells. Immunotherapy is a relatively

new and somewhat experimental, but potentially promising technique.

5. hormone therapy--Adrenocortisotrophic hormones (Cortisone and ACTH)
   may be used as an additive or suppressive treatment. For the last
   25 years, sex hormones have been used as an additive treatment
   in breast cancer and endometrial cancer in females and cancer of
   the prostate in males.

Each of these treatment methods and possible complications is presented
in greater detail in A Comprehensive Approach to Rehabilitation of the
Cancer Patient,[15] the companion to this text. Treatment procedures described
in this section have been presented primarily from a medical standpoint;
patient needs, concerns, and anxieties have been omitted. The patient's
interaction with physicians, nurses, physical therapists, medical social
service workers, and other members of the health care team* has not been
included because patient care is, in essence, "the art and the science" of
medicine, a subject much too broad to discuss here. However, it must be
pointed out that team members need to make every effort to see that the
patient and his immediate family: (1) understand the diagnosis, (2) are
kept informed of the steps in the treatment procedures, and (3) are aware
of the prognosis or possible outcome. When the patient and his family are
well informed, patient cooperation and communication are enhanced, and
team members' effectiveness and efficiency are increased.

Prognosis

In general, although the cancer patient's prognosis is guarded, there

---

* occupational therapist, enterostomal therapist, speech therapist,
  prosthetist/orthotist, vocational counselor, clinical psychologist,
  dietitian, inhalation therapist, hospital chaplain, and others.

is hope for increased, albeit uncertain survival time, and thought and effort have been turned to the "quality" of that survival.[4] The "quality of survival" is essentially what rehabilitation is all about. The quality of survival includes not only recovery from the extent and treatment of cancer, but also the general physical condition of the client five to ten years later. What is the patient like in five or ten years? Is he gainfully employed, or is he bedfast without energy and motivation?[3]

Influencing the quality of survival are the patient's (1) general health, (2) functional ability, (3) pain, (4) attitude, (5) economic status, and (6) physical condition.[4] Each of these aspects should be considered separately as well as in combination with other factors becasue of the difficulty in assessing quality of survival. Followup and rehabilitation are important factors both in prognosis and quality of survival. The "Suggested Reading" section at the end of this chapter contains references on both treatment of the cancer patient and on rehabilitation.

Safeguards

The following safeguards have been recommended by the American Cancer Society:

1. lung--reduction and ultimate elimination of cigarette smoking.
2. colon-rectum--proctoscopic exam and colonoscopy as routine in annual checkup for those over 40 years of age.
3. breast--self-examination as monthly female practice.
4. uterus--pelvic examination and Pap test for all women at risk, i.e., women who have begun active sex relations and for:
   a. women over age 35.
   b. woman who has never had a child.

    c. woman who bore her first child after age 25.

    d. women whose mothers or sisters had breast cancer.

    e. women who experienced early menarche and/or late menopause.

5. skin--avoidance of excessive sun.

6. oral--wider practice of early detection measures; avoidance of tobacco.

7. basic--regular physical examination for all adults.

Control of Cancer

The American Cancer Society is a volunteer health organization dedicated to the control and eradication of cancer. The major activities of the 2 million volunteers are (1) to bring life-saving information to their neighbors in the most effective way and (2) to raise funds to fight cancer.

The society's research program is directed toward (1) etiology, (2) pathogenesis, and (3) therapy. The main focus is on determining the cause of cancer and finding more effective ways to treat cancer through advances in surgery, radiation, chemotherapy, and immunotherapy.

The National Cancer Act

A National Cancer Act, passed by Congress in December 1971, was designed to strengthen the National Cancer Institute and to carry out more effectively the national effort against cancer. In September 1972, a Cancer Control Program was developed within the institute for the purpose of "cooperating with . . . health agencies in the diagnosis, prevention, and treatment of cancer."[7]

Reinforcement and Review

1.33 Match the diagnostic procedure on the left with the site or part of the body for which the procedure is used:

1. xeroradiography
2. "Pap" smear
3. arteriography
4. sigmoidoscopy

__ 1. breast
__ 2. cervix, lung, and mouth
__ 3. brain, kidney, liver, heart, and adrenal gland.
__ 4. rectum

1.34 According to Cobb, professionals involved in developing the treatment plan include:

1. _____

2. _____

3. _____

4. _____

5. _____

6. _____

1.35 Treatment plans must take into consideration the _____ and _____ status of the patient.

1.36 In all treatment of all cancer patients, the critical factor is:

_____

1.37 List four basic factors on which treatment methods depend:

1. _____

2. _____

3. _____

4. _____

1.38 In what ways may cancer be treated?

1. _____

2. _____

3. _____

4. _____

5. _____

1.39 Specific aspects related to the quality of survival include:

1. appearance
2. general health
3. intelligence
4. functional ability
5. communicativeness

6. physical condition
7. economic status
8. attitude
9. recreational activities
10. pain

1.40 According to Cobb, the quality of survival includes:

1. general status of the patient for the first year only.
2. status of the patient 5 to 10 years following treatment.
3. only his immediate concerns such as health and comfort.
4. employment at a meaningful job.
5. only ability to walk.

1.41 Specific safeguards for women recommended by the American Cancer Society are:

1. _____

2. _____

1.42 Specific safeguards for men and women recommended by the American Cancer Society are:

1. _____

2. _____

3. _____

(Complete your answer on the next page)

4. _____

5. _ _____

1.43 The American Cancer Society's goals are:

_____ and _____

1.44 The major activities of the American Cancer Society volunteers are:

_____ and _____

Answers to Questions 1.33 - 1.44

1.33 xeroradiography--breast, "Pap" smear--cervix, lung, and mouth,
arteriography--brain, kidney, liver, heart, and adrenal gland.
sigmoidoscopy--rectum.

1.34 surgeon, radiotherapist, internist or family physician, pathologist,
psychologist or psychiatrist, rehabilitation counselor.

1.35 physical and emotional.

1.36 quality of survival.

1.37 (1) particular characteristics of cancer (kind, aggressiveness, and
predictability). (2) therapeutic procedure. (3) cure rate. (4) patient's health.

1.38 surgery, radiotherapy, chemotherapy, immunotherapy, hormone therapy
(or any combination).

1.39 general health, functional ability, physical condition, economic
status, attitude, and pain. Other aspects may be included.

1.40 2 and 4.

1.41 monthly breast self-examination, Pap test (recommended every 6 - 12
months.)

1.42 reduce cigarette smoking, annual proctoscopic exam and colonoscopy
for persons over 40, avoidance of excessive sun, oral examination,
regular physical examination.

1.43 the control and eradication of cancer.

1.44 providing information on cancer and raising funds to fight cancer.

Definitions

1. alkylating agents--compounds that affect tumor cells in much the same way
    as irradiation; some of them produce full but temporary remission in
    chronic leukemia. These compounds include nitrogen mustard, triethylene
    malamine (TEM), and triethylene thiophosphoramide (Thio-TEPA).[5]

2. antimetabolites--compounds which interfere with tumor metabolism by
    substituting a metabolic analogue for an essential amino acid and cause
    remission in patients with leukemia. Some of these compounds are Aminop-
    terin[R] and Methotrexate[R].[5]

3. benign--not malignant.

4. deoxyribonucleic acid (DNA)--a nucleic acid found in all living cells;
    on hydrolysis it yields adenine, guanine, cytosine, thymine, deoxyribose,
    and phosphoric acid.

5. en bloc--in a lump or as a whole.

6. epidemiology--a research approach to the origins of disease which is based
    on observation rather than on experimentation. Descriptive epidemiology
    deals with the distribution of disease by such variables as sex, age,
    race, geographic distribution, and socioeconomic status. Analytical
    epidemiology is used to test ideas about etiology.

7. histologic--pertaining to the minute structure, composition, and function
    of tissues.

8. incidence--the number of new cases per unit of time in a defined popula-
    tion (usually based on 100,000 population).

9. keratosis--any horny growth such as a wart or callosity.

10. lesion--any pathological or traumatic discontinuity of tissue or loss
    of function of a part.

11. leukoplasia--a disease marked by the development of white, thickened patches on the mucous membrane of the cheeks, gums, or tongue. This disease is common in smokers and sometimes becomes malignant.

12. malignant--tending to produce death or deterioration.

13. metastasis--new tumor growth started by spreading of malignant cells from the primary site to a location in the body via blood vessels or lymphatic channels.[9]

14. pathogenesis--the development of morbid conditions or of disease.

15. radiographic--use of radioactivity to make records or photographs.

16. staging--a classification system which facilitates quantification of the extent of disease. Three major components in the quantification process are (1) definition of primary site of tumor, (2) lymph node involvement, (3) the spread of disease, or metastases. The abbreviated form is T (tumor), N (lymph node), and M (metastases).

Other Important Words Not Used In This Chapter But Related To Cancer:

1. biopsy--the removal of a section of body tissue of varying size for microscopic examination for the diagnosis or prognosis of disease.

2. neoplasm--new growth, and usually is considered a more precise term for tumor. This growth could be benign or malignant.

3. prevalence--total number of cases in a given population, which includes old and new cases.

36

References

1. American Cancer Society. <u>A cancer source book for nurses</u>. New York: American Cancer Society, Inc., 1975.

2. American Cancer Society. '75 Cancer facts and figures. New York: American Cancer Society, Inc., 1974.

3. Cobb, A.B. Medical and psychological problems in the rehabilitation of the cancer patient. In A.B. Cobb (Ed.), <u>Special problems in rehabilitation</u>. Springfield, Ill.: Charles C Thomas, 1974.

4. Cobb, A.B. (Ed.). <u>Special problems in rehabilitation</u>. Springfield, Ill.: Charles C Thomas, 1974.

5. Clark, R.L., & Cumley, R.W. (Eds.). <u>The book of health</u> (3rd ed.). New York: Van Nostrand Reinhold Co., 1973.

6. Craytor, J.K., & Fass, M.L. <u>The nurse and the cancer patient</u>. Philadelphia: J.B. Lippincott, 1970.

7. Edwards, M.H. In L.W. Green (Ed.), <u>Proceedings of the conference on cancer public education, July 31 - August 3, 1973</u>. San Francisco: Society for Public Health Education, Inc., 1973. (Health Education Monograph No. 36).

8. Emerson, G., & Phillips, C. Lung cancer. In P. Rubin (Ed.), <u>Clinical oncology for medical students and physicians</u> (4th ed.). New York: American Cancer Society, 1974.

9. Glossary prepared for Cancer training programs for occupational and physical therapists, Contract NO1-CN-45051, October, 1974.

10. Mountain States Tumor Institute. <u>What everyone should know about cancer</u>. Greenfield, Mass.: Channing L. Bete, 1971.

11. Oken, D. What to tell cancer patients: study of medical attitudes. <u>J.A.M.A.</u>, 1961, <u>175</u>, 1120-1128.

12. Potter, D.S. Specific problems related to the age of the child. In <u>Proceedings of the national conference on cancer nursing</u>. New York: American Cancer Society, Inc., 1974.

13. Richards, V. <u>Cancer: the wayward cell</u>. Berkeley: The University of California Press, 1972.

14. Rubin, P. (Ed.). <u>Clinical oncology for medical students and physicians</u> (3rd ed.). New York: American Cancer Society, 1971.

15. Smith, E.A. <u>A comprehensive approach to rehabilitation of the cancer patient</u>. (A publication of The University of Texas Health Science Center at Houston, Division of Continuing Education, 1975).

16. Spratt, J.S. Your behavior and cancer. Missouri Medicine, 1974, pp. 22A - 24.

17. Terry, R. Pathology of cancer. In P. Rubin (Ed.), Clinical oncology for medical students and physicians (4th ed.). New York: American Cancer Society, 1974.

Suggested Readings

Alcohol and the cancer connection. Medical World News, August 2, 1974, p. 21.

Brooks, M. The cancer story. New York: A.S. Barnes and Co., 1973.

Cunningham, C.J., Watson, F.R., Spratt, J.S., & Hahn, R.C. Behavioral sciences and cancer. Missouri Medicine, 1971, pp. 896-904.

Dial Access System. Makes available tapes on specific neoplastic disease problems. Health practitioners in the Southern Medical Association may use this cancer education service without charge by dialing the appropriate number: (1) Houston physicians dial 790-1683, (2) Texas physicians dial 1-800-392-3917, (3) all other physicians dial 1-800-231-6970.

Graham, S., & Schneiderman, M. Social epidemiology and the prevention of cancer. Preventive Medicine, 1972, 1, 371-380.

Healey, J.E., Jr. (Ed.). Ecology of the cancer patient. Washington, D.C.: Interdisciplinary Communication Associates, Inc., 1970.

Izsak, F.C., & Medalie, J.H. Comprehensive followup of carcinoma patients. J. Cron. Dis., 1971, 24, 179-191.

Chapter 2

UNDERSTANDING THE PATIENT WITH CANCER

The major components involved in a psychosocial approach to the study
of cancer are: (1) the patient and (2) the patient's environment, which
includes members of the health care team and the family and the physical
setting of the hospital, the clinic, or the home. The relationships between
cancer, the patient, and the patient's environment are complex. One way of
representing these dynamic multifaceted relationships is illustrated below.

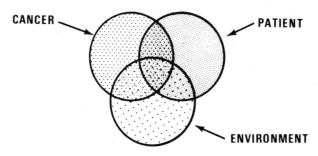

FIGURE 1

The interrelationship of these major components is entirely dependent
on the unique interaction between the patient, cancer, and the environment
at a given point in time. (Information on cancer was presented in Chapter 1;
this chapter will deal with the patient, and briefly, with the environment.)
Although the hospital or home environment may be relatively constant and
predictable, the patient's physical and psychological status and his understanding of his disease are subject to change. The accurate identification
and effective handling of changes in the patient's status and in his environment are of major significance.

The Patient

Important factors in understanding the patient with cancer are: (1) needs, (2) perceptions of the diagnosis of cancer, (3) reactions to the diagnosis of cancer, (4) adjustment to the diagnosis of cancer, (5) beliefs and attitudes, (6) identification of general and specific objectives, (7) motivation, and (8) attitude and behavior change. Each of these aspects is discussed in considerable detail in the following pages.

The patient with cancer faces a traumatic life-threatening situation, as the diagnosis of cancer is frequently associated with death. Whether the threat of death is real or imaginary, tremendous emotional strain is placed on the patient and on his family. The potential for debilitation and uncertainty of outcome is considered to be higher in the cancer patient than in the majority of patients with other diagnoses. Understandably, the cancer patient's problems exceed those of other patients in: (1) intensity, (2) frequency, and (3) duration. In addition, his ability to effectively mobilize his physical and emotional resources is frequently reduced. Since physical needs are usually given first attention, emotional needs may be considered of secondary importance. The primary physician, specialists, and other team members are usually too involved with the medical aspects of survival to attend to the patient's need for understanding and acceptance.

The pervasiveness of the diagnosis of cancer permeates the patient's very existence. The disease has many associated unconscious meanings and fantasies.[14] In many instances, cancer infiltrates the person's body, while thoughts of cancer infiltrate and occupy his mind. Since the patient can not be separated from his disease or his thoughts, it is necessary to consider the interaction of cancer and the patient. Most important aspects

relate to the patient's: (1) physical needs, (2) personal needs, (3) interpretation of the diagnosis of cancer, (4) reactions to the diagnosis, and
(5) adjustment--physical and emotional.

Needs

The cancer patient's needs are not unique. In wrestling with the diagnosis of cancer, the patient experiences certain persistent needs which
can often be determined by simply taking the time to find out what they are.
Whether these needs are met depends on the individual, the various aspects
of his disease, and his interaction with his surrounding environment. Specific needs which have been identified include:

1. needs related to physiology, safety, security, belongingness, and
   self-actualization, as outlined by Maslow.[13]

2. need to develop (as described by Erikson[5]):

    a. hope--enables people to believe and trust in themselves, in
       others, and in the future. Hope is an essential virtue of adult-
       hood, and an adult without hope will not survive.

    b. will--determination to exercise free choice as well as self-
       restraint in making decisions.

    c. purpose--a realistic goal which is related to what can be
       achieved and what cannot be achieved.

    d. competence--is the free exercise of dexterity and intelligence
       in the completion of tasks which are needed by society.

    e. fidelity--ability to freely enter into and to sustain pledged
       loyalties in relationships with other people.

    f. love--the greatest of all human virtues and the dominant virtue
       of the universe. Adult love is the mutuality of mates and

partners in a shared identity through an experience of finding

oneself, as one loses oneself in another.

    g. care--extending of solicitude and concern to other persons.

    h. wisdom--ability to view mankind and life itself in some perspec-

       tive, which may be short-range or long-range.

3. need to be an individual with rights, privileges, and some measure

of control over own destiny.

4. need to see self as whole person having the same needs and desires

as other fully functioning persons.

5. need to express emotions. Prevention of the expression of emotions

delays stress reactions, or reactions to grief, both of which are

necessary to the maintenance of emotional equilibrium.

6. need to have illness understood and to be able to talk about it.

7. need to have goals that are realistic, rewarding, and attainable.

These goals will differ depending on the physical and emotional

status of the patient, motivation, and level of expectation.

Patients' Perceptions of the Diagnosis of Cancer

The diagnosis of cancer means different things to different people.
The diagnosis will be much more devastating, for example, to persons whose
physical appearance and earning capacity are severely affected than to those
persons who are not similarly affected. The diversity of interpretations
and reactions is based on the following assumptions:

1. Most patients want to know if they have cancer.[2]

2. All patients with malignant disease have some awareness of it.[6]

3. The majority of patients understand something about their treat-

ment and know that a given form of treatment is associated with malignant disease.[6]

Since patients' perceptions of cancer are highly individualized,[2] interpretation depends on personality make-up, usual reactions to stress, customary methods of adjustment (which include use of ego defense mechanisms), interpersonal relationships, and the environment.

Some of the frequently occurring perceptions reported by cancer patients are:

1. extreme and prolonged pain and suffering.[2,6,9] A chronic, disabling, and unpleasant illness.[7]

2. rejection.[3,6]

3. physical isolation[3,6] and emotional isolation.[6]

4. disfigurement,[9] body mutilation or change in body image[1] and body function.[9]

5. not belonging.[16]

6. fear.[8,14]

7. not being wanted and loved.[6]

8. helplessness and awareness of lack of control over the disease.[6]

9. an extreme threat to existing lifelong patterns of adaptation which renders the course of development incalculable.[2]

10. an affront to masculinity or feminininity when eyes, limbs, breasts or genital organs are affected.[8]

11. certain death.[9,14]

Reinforcement and Review

2.1 The diagnosis of cancer is often associated with _____.

2.2 The cancer patient's physical and emotional problems exceed those of other patients in:

_____, _____, and _____.

2.3 Name what you feel to be the four most important aspects of understanding and managing the patient with cancer.

1. _____

2. _____

3. _____

4. _____

2.4 Which three of the needs specified by Maslow are most important to the cancer patient?

_____, _____, and _____

2.5 Which three of the needs specified by Erickson are most important to the cancer patient?

_____, _____, and _____

2.6 Four other vitally important needs are:

_____, _____, _____, and

_____

2.7 Interpretations and reactions are based on which of the following assumptions? Circle the correct response(s).

1. Most patients want to know if they have cancer.
2. Patients with malignant disease seldom are aware of it.
3. Patients know very little about their treatment.
4. Patients usually know that a given form of treatment is associated with malignant disease.
5. Diagnosis of cancer means different things to different people.

2.8 What major factors influence patients' perceptions of cancer?

      1.   _____

      2.   _____

      3.   _____

      4.   _____

2.9 List 5 of the most frequently occurring perceptions reported by cancer patients:

      1.   _____

      2.   _____

      3.   _____

      4.   _____

      5.   _____

Answers to Questions 2.1 - 2.9

2.1 threat of death. The current mortality rate of persons diagnosed as having cancer is 2 out of 3. This rate is decreasing steadily because of scientific advances in early detection, diagnosis, and treatment. Patients and health care team members are facing the diagnosis, treatment, and rehabilitation of cancer patients with increasing optimism. One of the objectives of the Cancer Control Program mentioned in Chapter 1 is to provide increased opportunities for public education concerning all aspects of cancer.

2.2 intensity, frequency, duration. There is some feeling that cancer patients are unique because of the possible long-term effects of the disease. However, many cancers, such as skin cancer, pose no threat to life whatsoever.

2.3 physical needs, personal needs, understanding of his diagnosis, reactions to diagnosis, and adjustment. Other needs may be equally appropriate, but the patients' needs and his understanding of his diagnosis are extremely important.

2.4 Your choice depends on your individual interests and priorities, but security and belonging are very important to the cancer patient.

2.5 Your choice depends on your own interests, but hope, purpose, and love are of particular significance. Purpose is especially important in rehabilitation. A definition of love slightly different from Erikson's is: when the happiness of another person is as important to one as one's own happiness or security.

2.6 need to be an individual, to see one's self as a whole person, to express emotions, and to have realistic goals. All of these needs are particularly important in rehabilitation of the cancer patient.

2.7 1, 4, and 5. 3 may be true in instances in which information is withheld for various reasons.

2.8 Personality make-up, adjustment, environmental factors, interpersonal relationships are generally considered to be of major importance.

2.9 Any of the 11 previously listed are correct. However, the most frequently reported ones are: extreme and prolonged pain and suffering, not belonging, physical and emotional isolation, death, and fear.

Reactions to the Diagnosis of Cancer

Patients' individualized reactions to the diagnosis of cancer are frequently influenced by situational factors such as immediate environment, daily pressures, team members, family, and physical well-being. The ethnic and social milieus in which persons are reared and live affect their perceptions of potentially painful experiences. However, there is commonality regarding initial reactions, establishment of adaptive patterns, and methods of preserving emotional integrity. Some of the most frequently occurring reactions are:

1. "stunned," "dizzy," "dazed," "numb all over," "unreal," "like receiving a heavy blow on the head," "rendered speechless," and a general feeling of depersonalization.[15]

2. feelings of hopelessness, apathy, anxious suspicion, burning hostility, wary intrigue, susceptibility to rumor, gullibility to charlatans, response to drug overdose, and superstition.[15]

3. feelings of guilt,[16] self-blame,[2] and feelings that one is being punished for something he has done wrong.[8]

4. preservation of emotional integrity through repression, suppression, denial,[6,9] fantasy, delusion-hallucination formation,[2] withdrawal,[16] and projection of blame.[2]

5. general disruption of adaptive patterns which require a massive reorganization of the patients' resources and a major shift in the internal or subjective system of priorities.[2] Patients may use any one of a variety of emergency or adaptational defensive techniques which lend a sense of mastery and permit the continuation of functioning.[2]

6. ongoing anxiety and uncertainty.[6]

7. conscious avoidance.

8. preoccupation with the disease.

9. complaints, constant calling for nurses, etc.[10]

10. fear of speaking openly about cancer.

The adaptational techniques of many of the social and cultural sub-groups may be similar, but the rules of expression and communication which are expressed above vary significantly.[2] There are also great individual differences in the extent to which patients can pursue their fears. In most cases, patients can handle fears in small doses.[9]

Fears first occur when a person either suspects that he has something wrong with him or when he recognizes one of the early warning signs of cancer. Despite early warning signs, there is often a delay in seeking treatment. Delay seems to be attributable to some defect in the processing of information at hand, or in Gestalt terms, failure of closure. Although the patient may have a vague awareness that something is wrong, he may not be able to describe anything but vague symptoms. In some instances, the patient is able to recognize symptoms and seek medical advice.

Defensive maneuvers used by the patient are: (1) avoidance--the patient overlooks the lesion, (2) suppression--the lesion is noticed and dismissed, and (3) denial--the significance is suspected but dismissed.[15] A variation in the denial pattern is "destiny neurosis." The patient is aware of the existence of the problem, but reacts with a conviction that "fate has willed it" and becomes resigned to his disease.[15] Patients may abandon themselves to chance and wait for a "magical" intervention.

In the attempt to adapt to the different environmental situations

which occur following the discovery of a malignant lesion, patients have
demonstrated almost the whole spectrum of <u>ego defense mechanisms</u> that have
been observed in the neurotic patient.[4] Additional information on ego
defense mechanisms and on <u>neurotic</u> and <u>psychotic behavior</u> is presented in
Coleman. Coleman's Classification of Abnormal Reaction Patterns is presented in the appendix.

Patients use defense mechansism to defend themselves against fear
and anxiety and also to carry out constructive adaptations to their problems.
The most frequently used mechanisms are: (1) suppression, (2) denial,
(3) dissociation, (4) identification, (5) regression, and (6) sublimation.[15]
Sources for definitions for each of the following defensive mechanisms are
from Coleman's psychology text and from cancer literature.[15]

1. suppression (or <u>repression</u>)--deliberately preventing painful or
    dangerous thoughts from entering consciousness.[4]

2. denial--protecting the self from unpleasant reality by refusal to
    perceive or face it, often by escapist activities such as preoc-
    cupation with other things.[4] Although the cancer patient suspects
    he has cancer, he dismisses the possibility.

3. dissociation--protecting the self by splitting into observer and
    actor, with a sense of confining one's identity to the observing
    part of oneself.[15]

4. identification--increasing feelings of worth by identifying self
    with a person or institution of illustrious standing.[4] Patients
    may identify with a patient they have previously known who had the
    same sort of illness. Through this economic way of handling infor-
    mation, they do not have to puzzle out the possible future course

of the illness, as they have all the predictions all worked out in terms of past experience; i.e., the patient plays a role.[15]

5. regression--retreating to an earlier developmental level involving fewer natural responses and usually a lower level of aspiration.[4] Patients may give up much of their freedom and independence of action in forming a dependent relationship to a physician who may be interpreted as a parent.[15]

6. sublimation--gratifying or working off frustrated sexual desires in nonsexual activities.[4] Although this occurrence is rare, the patient constructs an image of the family group without him, and on the basis of this construction, spends his remaining time working toward strengthening the family unit.[15] The patient may develop plans to be followed by family members after his death, help build up morale, family togetherness, etc., with the overall intent of furthering family relationships.

Adjustment to the Diagnosis of Cancer

The physical status of the patient is a major variable in the adjustment process. Adjustment may be said to have occurred when an individual is capable of functioning within his personal, social, and vocational potential.[2] Few patients can initially accept the diagnosis of cancer with intelligent, controlled anxiety. However, an intelligent approach assists the patient in resisting the onslaught of the disease by cooperating with the physician in the treatment process. Debilitating anxiety is alleviated by converting it to a controlled energy which may be mobilized to combat the disease.

The prime factors in the adjustment process are: (1) beliefs and

attitudes, (2) identification of specific, attainable objectives, (3) motivation, and (4) change. While these factors relate primarily to patients,
they may also apply to team members, family, and friends.

Beliefs and Attitudes

All beliefs and attitudes about disease, regardless of their derivation,
offer evidence that illness is both a social and a biological phenomenon.
Beliefs and attitudes can be particularly helpful in deciphering the complex-
ities of emotion and behavior and in providing clues to psychological management.[2] For example, there is some indication that the psychological
state of the cancer patient may be a factor in what is called "host resistance" or "host acquiescence" to cancer.[6,8] Additional information on
beliefs and attitudes and their relationship to the rehabilitation process
is presented in Chapter 3 of A Comprehensive Approach to Rehabilitation of
the Cancer Patient,[17] the companion to this text.

Reinforcement and Review

2.10 List 5 of the most frequent reactions to the diagnosis of cancer.

    1. _____

    2. _____

    3. _____

    4. _____

    5. _____

2.11 Delay in seeking medical treatment may be attributed to:

    1. _____

    2. _____

2.12 Defense mechanisms used by the patient are:

        _____, _____, and _____.

2.13 Define each of the following:

    1. suppression--_____

        _____

    2. denial--_____

        _____

    3. dissociation--_____

        _____

    4. identification--_____

        _____

    5. regression--_____

        _____

    6. sublimation--_____

    (Complete your answer on the next page.)

_____

2.14 The six most frequently used defense mechanisms are:

1. _____   4. _____

2. _____   5. _____

3. _____   6. _____

2.15 In addition to physical variables, what three major factors contribute
      to the patient's adjustment to the diagnosis of cancer?

1. _____

2. _____

3. _____

2.16 What are the 4 most important factors in the adjustment process?

1. _____

2. _____

3. _____

4. _____

2.17 There is evidence that illness should be considered from a

_____ and _____ standpoint.

2.18 The psychological state of the cancer patient may be a factor in

_____.

Answers to Questions 2.10 - 2.18

2.10 All ten previously listed are frequent reactions, but the most common are: stunned feeling, guilt, disruption of adaptive patterns, anxiety, and fear of speaking openly about cancer.

2.11 (1) inability to describe specific symptoms and (2) use of defensive maneuvers, or defense mechanisms.

2.12 avoidance, suppression, and denial.

2.13 (1) Suppression--preventing painful or dangerous thoughts from entering consciousness, (2) Denial--protecting the self from unpleasant reality by refusal to face it, often through escapist activities, (3) Dissociation--protecting the self by splitting into observer and actor, with a sense of confining one's identity to the observing part of the self, (4) Identification--increasing feelings of worth by identifying self with person or institution of illustrious standing, (5) Regression--retreating to an earlier developmental level involving less natural responses and usually a lower level of aspiration, (6) Sublimation--gratifying or working off frustrated sexual desires in nonsexual activities.

2.14 (1) suppression, (2) denial, (3) dissociation, (4) identification, (5) regression, and (6) sublimation.

2.15 (1) personal, (2) vocational, (3) social.

2.16 Major factors are: (1) beliefs and attitudes, (2) specific objectives, (3) motivation, and (4) change. You may list others which you consider equally important; however, each one should be sufficiently broad and capable of being supported.

2.17 social and biologic.

2.18 host resistance or host acquiescence to cancer.

Identification of General and Specific Objectives

Before developing any specific objectives with the patient, it is necessary to (1) establish a good relationship with him and (2) thoroughly understand facts about his diagnosis, prognosis, and treatment. Since the most effective factor in the care of a particular patient with cancer is his relationship with the physician who has taken care of him through the course of his illness, there must be a considerable effort to maintain this relationship.[8] The physician-patient relationship can be used as a framework around which good relationships with team members can be built. Once team members have been accepted by the patient, good relationships which have been established will "spill over" to others and enhance their effectiveness in patient care.

By encouraging the patient to direct himself toward responsibility for his own behavior, or "helping the patient to help himself," you will help him to practice constructive behavior, such as eating meals at a table rather than in bed. If the patient is mobile, he can be encouraged to do other tasks, such as helping a patient in the adjoining room. By systematically involving the patient in helping, recreational, and vocational activities, you will encourage him to decide on his own daily routine; he will thus develop goals and responsibilities that are intrinsically his. When these behaviors become clearly established, performance objectives (for example, "patient gets out of bed to eat meals") and the level of acceptable performance (for example, "patient eats all meals out of bed") can readily be determined.

In setting up behavioral objectives, the following steps are recommended: (1) identify observable action, (2) describe observable performance,

(3) describe important conditions under which performance is to occur, (4) specify the criteria by which performance is to be measured, and (5) state the level of acceptable performance. These objectives may be adapted to assessment of patients' adjustment.[12]

Specific objectives to be identified relate to all phases of patient care and welfare. By helping the patient understand his feelings and cope with the present, team members can greatly facilitate the identification of objectives and needs. These needs can be rank ordered once they are expressed and discussed. Typical needs may relate to dependency, dissatisfaction, emotional and adjustment problems, or to personality and family. While the needs of cancer patients are not unique, the priorities placed on needs and the ways in which they are to be met may differ significantly.

Patient behaviors can be observed directly and/or pertinent information can be obtained from team members, other patients, family, medical records, etc. These behaviors can be discussed with the patient, as once he knows team members are interested in him, he may approach them for assistance.

Measuring or quantifying performance may be difficult, but standards can be developed. Your own experience and intuition and the expertise of other team members will enable you to construct realistic standards for most patients.

Motivation

A traditional definition of motivation includes: (1) the process of arousing actions, (2) sustaining the activity in progress, and (3) regulating the pattern of activity. Motivation may also be defined in terms of competence or the person's capacity to interact effectively with his environment.[18] Motives may be considered synonymous with needs or drives. Although there are many theories of motivation, some of which are conflicting, the assumption that all patients are motivated is basic. However, not all patients reach for the same goals. Motivation is inferred from behavior and is often confused with the method of achievement instead of achievement itself.

Once the patient is involved in daily routines which include not only helping himself, but others as well, the obvious assumption is that he is motivated. Factors which tend to reduce motivation are: (1) dependency, (2) dissatisfaction, (3) difficulty in overcoming emotional and adjustment problems, as exemplified by inability to adjust to a routine or to identify with other persons (patients, team members, and family), (4) personal, family, or job-related problems, and (5) a progressively deteriorating physical condition.

Motivation is a highly individual matter because the variables influencing motivation vary with the patient's mood, how well he feels, his interpersonal relationships, and many other factors. Motivation is difficult to measure, particularly in the hospital or clinic setting. If team members focus their approach to patient motivation on the integrity of the individual and on a concern for human dignity, patients will undoubtedly respond in a positive manner.

Attitude and Behavior Change

There are many ways in which attitude or behavior change may be effected, but change may occur very slowly. There are two basic ways of approaching behavior change: (1) overcoming resistance to change, which implies use of pressure, coercion, and possibly threat and (2) reducing resistance to change. The latter way is much superior, and typically consists of methods which: (1) involve the patient in discussions regarding proposed change, (2) allow for slow yet progressive change, and (3) employ effective two-way communication. Efforts to change or modify attitudes or behavior are most effective under the following circumstances:

1. when there is direct evidence that change is in order and the patient recognizes it. If a patient has an uncooperative attitude, is dissatisfied with his treatment, is depressed, etc., the probability of changing his behavior is decreased.

2. when change of behavior or attitude is determined to positively influence the effectiveness of treatment.

3. when new methods of treatment are to be used, or when the patient must accept and adjust to radical surgery such as amputation, mastectomy, etc.

Attitude or behavior change is most important when patient behavior is critical. Attempts at attitude change will not be successful unless the patient understands why it is important to change his behavior. When treatment procedures are involved, the patient is most likely to be concerned and willing to change his behavior.

Change is most readily accepted by the patient:

1. when some authority figure (physician, nurse, psychologist, physical therapist, social worker, or family member) whom the patient respects recommends the adoption of a new treatment method, counseling, exercise program, or vocational counseling, for example.

2. when the patient has been adequately prepared for or anticipates the intervention or change and is counseled on its possible effects and outcome. Change which challenges integrity, capableness,

status, and skills must be carefully presented to and discussed with the patient.

3. when there has been time to discuss the change with other patients experiencing similar treatment or problems and when there is an understanding that the change is in his best interests.

Change cannot be effective unless:

1. changed behavior or changed attitudes are reinforced by team members, family, and other persons. Reinforcement should be based on empathy and understanding.

2. the environment in which change occurs is supportive or conducive to changed behavior. If the patient changes his behavior, the hospital, home, or work environment must be planned in such a way that continuing support and incentives are provided.

3. patients are encouraged to be physically and mentally active and to exert these resources in maintaining their new behavior. Patients who remain active are certainly happier, better adjusted, and more likely to take an interest in life than those who are inactive.

4. patients are discouraged from preoccupation with their own problems and from viewing other persons' problems in terms of their own needs. Patients should be encouraged to develop constructive relationships with other patients and a continuing recognition of their own contributing role. For example, with the proper encouragement and supervision, patients may become involved in the care of other patients by carrying food trays, straightening bedcovers, writing letters, and many other helpful comforting activities.

Typical reactions of persons who resist change include: (1) negative attitudes, (2) anxiety, (3) resignation, (4) use of ego-defensive mechanisms such as projection, and (5) aggression. The magnitude of resistance can frequently be reduced by using a positive, logical approach to finding out the cause(s) of patient resistance and following procedures outlined to reduce resistance to change.

The Environment

The major components in the patient's environment are the physical setting and all persons with whom he has contact during all phases of treatment. The health care team members who are directly involved in patient care greatly influence his interpretation of and response to his environment.

The hospital is the physical setting that has the most impact on the cancer patient even though he may be frequently treated in an out-patient clinic. Although the structured, protected, sterile environment of the hospital is ideally suited to the optimization of patient care, the patient is expected to and usually does play a submissive, dependent role. In some instances, the patient must be shielded and protected from a potentially disruptive and unpredictable environment. On the other hand, patients who are encouraged by team members to achieve the goals of independence and self-care can do so only in an environment conducive to such activities.

An environment which fosters independence is one in which: (1) open and honest two-way communication between the patient and team members is encouraged, (2) the patient is assisted by team members in analyzing realistic goals, and (3) the patient is encouraged and/or allowed to become an active member of the health care team and perhaps even the leader.

Additional environmental variables are discussed in connection with the communication process, which is presented in Chapter 3. Personality characteristics and common modes of adjusting to the diagnosis of cancer and to hospitalization are discussed in Chapter 4. Information contained in these two chapters is considered basic to understanding the typical behavior of both cancer patients and team members in their unique and common environments.

Reinforcement and Review

2.19 Before developing specific objectives with the patient, what is nec-
      essary?

      1. _____

      2. _____

2.20 The most important relationship is that between the patient and the:

      _____.

2.21 Ways to get the patient involved in self-care include:

      1. _____

      2. _____

2.22 Major guidelines to be followed in setting up behavioral objectives
      include:

      1. _____

      2. _____

      3. _____

      4. _____

2.23 Define motivation using your own terms:

      _____

      _____

2.24 Factors which tend to reduce motivation are:

      1. _____

      2. _____

      3. _____

      4. _____

      (Complete your answer on the next page.)

5. _____

2.25 Patients are most likely to be motivated by methods which focus on

_____ and _____ .

2.26 What methods may be used to reduce resistance to change?

1. _____

2. _____

3. _____

2.27 When is change most readily accepted by patients?

1. _____

2. _____

3. _____

2.28 Change cannot be effective unless:

1. _____

2. _____

3. _____

4. _____

2.29 What are typical reactions of persons who resist change?

1. _____

2. _____

3. _____

4. _____

5. _____

2.30 List your typical individual reactions to proposed change:
(Use the next page to answer the question.)

1. _____

2. _____

3. _____

4. _____

5. _____

2.31 The major components in the patient's environment are:

1. _____

2. _____

2.32 Does the hospital environment unnecessarily restrict patients' activities which encourage independence?

___yes/___no. Why? _____

_____

2.33 What kind of physical environment fosters patient independence?

_____

_____

2.34 Can the hospital environment be changed?

___yes/___no. Please explain: _____

_____

_____

Answers to Questions 2.19 - 2.30

2.19 (1) establish a good relationship with him and (2) understand facts relative to his diagnosis, prognosis, and treatment.

2.20 physician. Other relationships may be just as meaningful to the patient, but the bond between patient and physician is very strong and basic.

2.21 (1) helping the patient to help himself and (2) getting the patient interested in various constructive activities.

2.22 Since you probably have some experience in establishing behavioral objectives, your wordings may be slightly different from those listed in the text. However, each objective must be stated in terms of patients' needs and expected outcomes of behavior. Good references are Mager.[11,12]

2.23 Many definitions are acceptable. Examples are: to move or to activate, initiate activity, a drive, a need, a force, an internal impetus behind behavior, and goal-directed behavior. Conscious and unconscious aspects of motivation should also be considered.

2.24 (1) dependency, (2) dissatisfaction, (3) difficulty in overcoming emotional and adjustment problems, (4) personal, family, or job-related problems, and (5) a progressively deteriorating physical condition. Many factors may reduce motivation. Only selected examples are listed above. Since motivation is such a complex process, determining major influencing factors is extremely difficult.

2.25 (1) the integrity of the individual and (2) a concern for human dignity. Other human relations approaches are possible, but the emphasis should be on patient priorities.

2.26 (1) Discuss the change with the patient, (2) allow for slow, yet progressive change, and (3) employ effective two-way communication. These are representative examples. Methods based on your own experience are equally appropriate.

2.27 (1) when a respected authority figure is involved in the change process, (2) when the patient is adequately prepared for possible changes, (3) when there has been time for discussion, and the patient understands the change is in his best interests.

2.28 (1) changed behavior is reinforced, (2) the environment is conducive or supportive of changed behavior, (3) patients are encouraged to be physically and mentally active, (4) patients are discouraged from being preoccupied with their own problems.

2.29 (1) negative attitudes, (2) anxiety, (3) resignation, (4) use of ego-defensive mechanisms such as projection, and (5) aggression.

2.30 Your choice is an individual matter. No answer is provided.

2.31 (1) physical setting and (2) team members.

2.32 The hospital has traditionally, yet realistically, placed certain limitations and restrictions on patient behavior. There is an increasing
emphasis on encouraging independence and self-care, both of which:
(1) reduce the length of hospitalization, (2) perceptibly decrease
the work load of team members, and (3) facilitate the whole process
of rehabilitation by motivating the patient to make every effort
possible to become independent as soon as realistically possible.

2.33 an environment in which: (1) there is open and honest two-way communication, (2) team members are willing and able to help the patient
achieve his desired goals, and (3) the patient is encouraged to act-
ively participate as a team member.

2.34 Hospital environments are very difficult to change, as organizational
structures are relatively rigid. However, it is possible to gradually
increase the openness of the atmosphere in a ward, unit, or floor of
a hospital by encouraging and continually reinforcing team members'
positive attitudes toward patient care and patient independence. All
change takes place slowly.

Definitions

1. acceptable performance-- through the process of measurement or evaluation, the level of performance is determined, and a comparison made with a norm (norm-referenced evaluation) or with an objective standard (criterion-referenced evaluation). Once the comparison has been made, a judgment (pass/fail, etc.) is made.[11]

2. attitude-- a predisposition to react in a certain way, a readiness to react, a determining tendency.

3. beliefs-- convictions, an acceptance of something as real, or accepted as true.

4. ego defense mechanisms-- reactions designed to maintain the individual's feelings of adequacy and worth rather than to cope directly with the stress situation. Such reactions are usually unconscious and reality distorting.[4]

5. emotional isolation-- psychological condition of being alone without any meaningful personal relationships.

6. health care team -- the following are considered to be most frequently involved in rehabilitation of cancer patients:

   <u>medicine</u>

   a. physician

   <u>nursing</u>

   b. nurse

   <u>Functional Restoration</u>

   c. maxillofacial prosthodontist
   d. occupational therapist
   e. physical therapist

   f. enterostomal therapist--R.N.
   g. prosthetist/orthotist
   h. speech therapist

   <u>Psychosocial and Vocational</u>

   i. vocational counselor
   j. medical social worker
   k. clinical psychologist
   l. dietitian
   m. inhalation therapist--R.N.
   n. hospital chaplain

7. intervention -- an intervening or coming between a person experiencing some crisis or stress situation and the source (situation or person) of the "atypical" or "unusual" behavior for the purposes of assisting the person experiencing the crisis or stressful situation. During the period in which the intervention is made, the therapist or "intervenor" may make suggestions, set examples, provide reassurance, give advice, or set forth prohibitions. Interventions should be insight-producing and motivate the patient to take the responsibility for his own behavior. Interventions should encompass both treatment and preventive aspects.

8. neurotic behavior or neurosis -- mild functional personality disorder in which there is no gross personality disorganization. The patient ordi-

narily does not require hospitalization.

9. performance objectives -- descriptions of objectives the person is expected to perform.

10. psychotic behavior or psychosis --severe personality disorder involving loss of contact with reality and usually characterized by delusions and hallucinations. Hospitalization is usually required.[4]

11. repression --preventing painful or dangerous thoughts and desires from entering consciousness without awareness of what is happening. Repression may also be considered to be selective forgetting. Suppression differs from repression in that the individual consciously "puts the idea out of his mind" and thinks of other things.[4]

References

1. Barckley, V. Grief, a part of living. Ohio's Health, 1968, 20, 34-38.

2. Bard, M. Clues to the psychological management of patients with cancer.
    Ann. N.Y. Acad. Sci., 1966, 125, 995-999.

3. Brennan, M.J. The cancer gestalt. Geriatrics, 1970, 25, 96-101.

4. Coleman, J.C. Abnormal psychology and modern life (3rd ed.). Chicago:
    Scott, Foresman, and Co., 1964.

5. Erikson, E.H. Human strength and the cycle of generations. Insight and
    responsibility. New York: W.W. Norton and Co., 1964.

6. Feder, S.L. Psychological considerations in the care of patients with
    cancer. Ann. N.Y. Acad. Sci., 1966, 125, 1020-1027.

7. Freireich, Emil J Death with dignity? The Cancer Bulletin, 1974, 26,
    110-114.

8. Greene, W.A. Psychological aspects of cancer. In P. Rubin (Ed.), Clinical
    oncology for medical students and physicians (3rd ed.). New York:
    American Cancer Society, 1971.

9. Heusinkveld, K.B. Cues to communication with the terminal cancer patient.
    Nursing Forum, 1972, 11, 105-113.

10. Klagsbrun, S.C. Communications in the treatment of cancer. Am. J. Nursing,
    1971, 71 (5), 944-948.

11. Mager, R.F. Measuring instructional intent. Belmont, California: Fearon
    Publishers, 1973.

12. Mager, R.F. Preparing instructional objectives. Belmont, California:
    Fearon Publishers, 1962.

13. Maslow, A.H. Motivation and personality. New York: Harper and Bros.,
    1954.

14. Oken, D. What to tell cancer patients: a study of medical attitudes.
    J.A.M.A., 1961, 175, 1120-1128.

15. Shands, H.C., Finesinger, J.E., Cobb, S., & Abrams, R.D. Psychological
    mechanisms in patients with cancer. Cancer, 1951, 4, 1159-1170.

16. Shepardson, J. A team approach to the patient with cancer. Am. J. of
    Nursing, 1972, 72 (3), 488-491.

17. Smith, E.A. A comprehensive approach to rehabilitation of the cancer
    patient. (A publication of The University of Texas Health Science
    Center at Houston, Division of Continuing Education, 1975).

18. White, R.W. Motivation reconsidered: the concept of competence. Psychol.
     Rev., 1959, 66, 297-333.

Chapter 3

COMMUNICATION

Communication involves a chain with at least three major links--a sender, a communication channel, and a receiver or listener.[14] Senders and receivers are most likely to be the cancer patient, his family, and members of the health care team. The channel is the medium through which communications are conveyed. Communication is frequently verbal, although it may be written (orders and charts) and nonverbal (gestures and facial expressions).

The communication process is complex. There are many general and specific factors which influence the effectiveness and efficiency of the process. Feedback, a vital component of the process, cannot be underestimated. Feedback provides the speaker or sender with information about his listener and also with specific data from his immediate environment. Information which is fed back to the speaker may cause him to reevaluate or modify his thought processes and behavior.

Major types of communications are: (1) cognitive information which is concerned primarily with facts about people, problems, events, and beliefs and (2) affective information which relates to individuals' feelings and emotions and to how persons feel about things.[4]

General Factors

Some of the general factors involved in the communication process are:

1. content of the communication, which may range from trivial to extremely important.

2. frequency--how often one communicates, or the number of times a certain topic is mentioned.

3. duration--the length of the communication.

4. distortion or misrepresentation, which may be attributed to the
   listener, the speaker (informant), or the communication channel.

5. level of complexity--the nature of the communication may not be
   readily understood because of complex terminology, language barriers,
   or other related variables.

The majority of communications revolve around the patient's diagnosis,
treatment, and prognosis. The cancer patient is continually alert for information pertinent to his immediate and future well-being and to the needs of
his family. Whether the patient hears, understands, accepts, and believes
the communication is a controversial matter, particularly when the information conveyed may be unpleasant, complex, or in conflict with previously
assimilated information. For example, the patient's anxiety level may be
so high that he does not hear what the physician or other team members
tell him regarding his diagnosis and/or prognosis.

Barriers to Communication

The most common barriers to effective communication are emotional ones.
The ego defense mechanisms of avoidance, denial, rejection, and repression
may be exhibited by cancer patients who desire (either consciously or unconsciously) to protect themselves from unpleasant communications. It is
natural that they avoid these unpleasant communications because these messages may convey life-threatening information.

Other barriers include depression, which may be exhibited through behavior ranging from passive avoidance to complete silence. Stage of disease
is integrally related to depression. A negative attitude, which may be
evidenced by anger, hostility, and aggression also prevents the free flow
of communication. A person in a highly anxious state may block out all

incoming communication. Communication skills will become sharpened as anxiety decreases.

Openness and willingness to communicate are greatly influenced by the patient's attitude toward the physician and the stage of his disease. Communication between physician and patient regarding the psychological impact of the disease and the patient's conception of the illness is impor- tant if the physician aspires to more than a mechanistic standard of medical management. Neglect in this area deprives the patient of an extremely valu- able source of emotional support and exposes him to potential delusions, conceptions, or experiences that are disruptive to his life's activities.[16]

The following commonly overlooked barriers may be overcome with effort and understanding by both the speaker and the listener:

1. age--A child may not know how to communicate or realize the impor- tance of communicating. The health care team may not perceive there is a need to communicate. Teenagers may think they are mis- understood and that no one (including their parents) cares about them. In their effort to be heroic, they may attempt to be com- pletely independent and to solve their own problems.

2. ethnic groups--Tradition may dictate that the patient be strong, stoic, brave, and self-reliant and not give in to his emotions.

3. dissonance in socio-cultural values--may decrease the rapport be- tween the physician and the patient, as background, expectations, and standards may be different. Each person or group has difficulty communicating with and understanding the other.

4. receptivity of the listener--Certain members of the team such as nurses and therapists may be in communication with the patient

more frequently than the physician. Patients may incorrectly

assume that the physician is too busy to answer their questions or

allay their fears. On the other hand, the physician may not

wish to disprove the stereotyped impression of an "overworked doctor"

that the patient holds in his mind.

5. semantics--Word meanings are subject to differential interpretation.
   Persons may be unfamiliar with the shades of meaning attached to
   certain words. It is only through contact with other persons that
   we begin to understand the usages and subtleties of certain words.

Factors Influencing Acceptance of Communications

Many factors influence the acceptance of communications. The following

factors apply to all persons, not just to cancer patients. Information

is more likely to be accepted if:

1. the communication is similar to that which the listener expects to
   hear.

2. the information is given by an authority figure (physician, nurse,
   medical social worker, parent, spouse, respected friend, etc.).

3. the listener is receptive to what is being communicated. This
   receptivity is influenced by:

   a. physical status of the listener--physical discomfort, auditory
      acuity, etc.

   b. psychological status of the listener--anxiety, depression, etc.

   c. mental set--whether the person is ready to listen.

   d. frame of reference, which in influenced by past, present, and
      future conditions such as sociocultural background, socioeconomic
      status, education, etc.

Acceptance of communication is a function of the subtle interplay of physical, psychological, and environmental factors. The effective communicator who uses repetition, selects the optimum time to speak or listen, or in some way optimizes the information exchange process, is frequently able to get his message across. Similarily, he is able to interpret messages sent by other persons.

Reinforcement and Review

3.1 The three major links in the communication process are:

_____, _____, and _____

3.2 The major factors involved in the communication process are:

_____, _____, and _____

3.3 One of the most essential components in the communication process is:

_____.

3.4 Based on your own experience, list three important functions of feed-back:

1. _____

2. _____

3. _____

3.5 The most common ego defense mechanisms which serve as barriers to effective communication are:

_____, _____, _____, and

_____

3.6 All of these barriers may be classified as:

_____

3.7 Major factors influencing the patient's openness and willingness to communicate are his attitude toward:

_____ and _____

3.8 What do you feel are the barriers to effective communication?

_____

_____

(Complete your answer on the next page.)

_____

_____

3.9 Considering the three major links in the communication process, draw a diagram illustrating the interrelationships between these links.

3.10 Add to your drawing the variables which influence the efficiency and effectiveness of the communication exchanged by the sender and the receiver. Variables should be consistent with your own professional training and your interpretation of potential problems experienced by patients and team members.

Answers to Questions 3.1 - 3.10

3.1 sender, receiver, and channel.

3.2 field of communication, content, distortion, and level of complexity
are probably the most important factors, although frequency and duration are common measurements.

3.3 feedback.

3.4 Your answer should include reference to the need for input of information from other persons so that the validity and reliability of the
information you communicate may be evaluated. Other persons use these
same procedures to clarify and to check on the information you are
communicating.

3.5 avoidance, denial, rejection, repression.

3.6 emotional.

3.7 his physician, his disease.

3.8 age, ethnic differences, dissonance in socio-cultural values, a
listener that is not receptive, and problems due to semantics.
You may not feel these are the most important barriers, but they are
the ones most frequently overlooked. They may never be overcome, but
with effort and understanding, open communication is definitely possible.

3.9 A typical representation may look like:
and
3.10

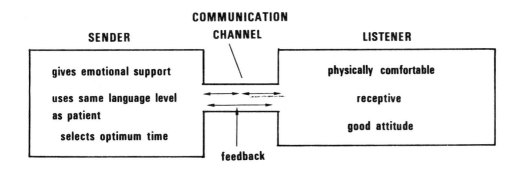

A more comprehensive drawing is presented at the end of the chapter.

What to Tell the Cancer Patient Regarding the Diagnosis

The one question continually faced by the health care team, but particularly by the physician, the nurse, and the medical social worker is "what to tell the cancer patient?" Should the patient who has a malignancy and is terminally ill be told the truth? If so, by whom? When should the patient be told?

The following approaches (not arranged in any specific order of importance) represent a summary of the current literature. Each guideline should be critically evaluated to determine its merits or limitations. Established practices may either support or conflict with the approaches presented below.

1. The patient should not be told anything until an histological diagnosis has been established.[18]

2. Although the patient may not wish to be informed of more of the situation than he asks or wants to know about, there may be times when knowing his exact status would be beneficial in terms of treatment and diagnosis.

3. A patient who is sick enough to die knows it without being told. [5,15]

4. A patient should not be told that he is dying. He will tell you he is dying when you dare to listen and when you are able to accept it.[13]

5. Patients should be told when they have a serious illness. The person telling them must allow for some hope and assure them that they will not be left alone.[13]

6. The issue is not simply "telling the truth," but never telling the patient anything patently untrue. The patient should never be

told anything that any member of the health care team would have to rescind and consequently cause disappointment.[5]

7. If directly confronted by the question, "Am I dying?" you may wish to inquire what he has been told, and why he directs the question to you. You could ask, "What do you think you have?" Patients rarely ask whether they are dying, particularly those who have a fair length of time to live.[8] In some instances, patients ask whether they are dying just to get your reaction and attention. However, whatever you tell them must be thought through very carefully. In general, no specific areas should be avoided if the patient wants to talk about them.

8. When a terminally ill cancer patient is told the medical facts about his illness, not all coping mechanisms are taken away. The patient can continue to function, as there is little risk that he will become psychotic,[8] or that he will take his own life.[8,15]

9. Telling a patient that his condition is hopeless is both cruel and technically incorrect.[19]

Studies (Kelly & Friesen,[11] Branch,[3] Samp & Curreri[17]) summarized by Oken[15] have revealed that approximately 87% of a total of 630 patients questioned want to know their diagnoses. However, the patient's wishes to be told their diagnoses did not always correspond with physicians' practices of revealing them. Factors contributing to the physicians' practices regarding disclosure of diagnoses were:

1. the belief that fatal illness is a major defeat.

2. the reaction that cancer connotes certain death.

3. the thought that the expectation of death insurmountably deprives

the patient of hope.

4. the belief that the patient's hope must be sustained and bolstered whenever possible.

According to Oken,[15] each physician uses his own preferred plan, select euphemisms, tactics, and views about the optimal time for discussions with patients. The degree of directness and the method of approach to the topic of death may vary, although some physicians have a set pattern. Some physicians tell patients the diagnosis when the prognosis is good; others tell the diagnosis when the prognosis is poor. In some instances, when patients are in far-advanced stages of illness, falsification occurs. For example, words such as "cancer" and "malignancy" are avoided; instead, words such as "lesion," "mass," "growth," or "tumor" and the like are used, sometimes in conjunction with false explicit statement that the process is benign.

There seems to be little evidence of a relationship between incidence of severe emotional problems (or even suicide) and the patient's knowledge of the diagnosis.[8,15] The real question is, "Can the patient stand not being told?" rather than, "Can the patient stand being told?" In general, the decision regarding disclosure of diagnosis by the physician is based primarily on the physician's intuitive understanding of the patient's concurrent experiences.[15]

Although the majority of communications may initially focus on the diagnosis, of equal or perhaps even greater importance are communications pertaining to (1) treatment, (2) side-effects, and (3) prognosis. The reader is referred to Chapter 2 of the companion text, A Comprehensive Approach to Rehabilitation of the Cancer Patient, for detailed information in each of these areas.

In some instances the patient has no conception of the nature or the extent of treatment. Team members seldom take the time to find out what the patient has been told even though it is not common to withhold information. Patients may be reluctant to ask questions because they feel the doctors or nurses are too busy to answer them or because they are afraid of showing their ignorance. The side effects of chemotherapy such as nausea, vomiting, and loss of appetite may, for example, be wrongly attributed to the spread of cancer. In such instances, the accompanying mental anguish and side-effects may have a more deleterious effect on the mental and physical welfare of the patient than the disease itself. Patients' ability to cope with the disease is greatly enhanced in an atmosphere in which there is free and open communication regarding all phases of treatment.

Communication Throughout the Course of Cancer

In the initial stage of cancer, communication is frequently direct and truthful. Once treatment starts, communication may be less open, and the patient may exhibit avoidance or denial behavior.[1] Sometimes patients want to share their experiences with someone but do not know whom to approach. This dilemma may result in later communication difficulties.

In the advancing stage, the patient seldom confronts his physician for information, but questions other team members about prognosis and treatment. Changes in the doctor-patient relationship result. The patient becomes passive, overnice, and uncomplaining,[2] and communication is minimized. The patient needs the physician's acceptance most during this time, but he may not be able to communicate his needs.

In the terminal stage, the dying patient needs communication and exchange with those around him more desparately than do other types of patients, yet as death approaches, communication becomes minimal, except in the area of the patient's anxieties.[1] A considerable number of terminal patients clearly display withdrawal or detachment.

The patient may use ego defense mechanisms as a means of preserving his integrity. He may, for instance, project blame for his illness on to the physician.[1] Other defense mechanisms may be rationalization and regression; these defenses make possible a facade of social acceptance which permits the patient to continue functioning.

Denial, which may occur in any stage, is the most prominent defense mechanism used by the dying patient. Through denial, the patient avoids open relationships with team members, family, and friends. He is frequently silent or uncommunicative, yet he indicates a need for continual support. On the other hand, the patient may develop a total acceptance of the nature and eventual ritual of illness without any appearance of anxiety.[7]

The patient who continues to deny that he has cancer selectively blocks himself off from all information regarding his disease. He consequently begins to feel isolated and rejected. The patient's feelings of rejection may be justified because the majority of persons may give up trying to communicate since they can not "get through" to him. Since denial is a poor avenue for emotional discharge, the patient is limited in the ways in which he may release tension. There is evidence to indicate that when the discharge of tension is blocked, mechanisms unfavorable to the patient's resistance to cancer may be encouraged.[5] Conversely, patients who have adequate avenues for the discharge of tension have a more favorable later course with cancer.

Since denial is not always beneficial, its use by the patient should be carefully monitored. While it may be easier for team members to support denial, the patient may interpret this support as reinforcement. If the pattern of denial appears to be firmly established, team members should consider whether some form of intervention would be appropriate. The intervention may be minor and consist of helping the patient to clarify his feelings on a specific issue, or it may be major and consist of one hour of counseling or psychotherapy. The patient's physical and psychological willingness must be critically evaluated before any intervention is planned. More harm may be done by confronting him with reality than by supporting denial, as denial and hope may be synonomous in the patient's mind. If hope is destroyed, the patient may have little reason for living. The patient may achieve satisfactory equilibrium by concentrating on treatment procedures and daily routines instead of focusing on the existence of the disease.

Prolonged anger and hostile behavior are relatively common among the chronically ill.[8] Patients' hostile behavior may be primarily attributed to: (1) team members' lack of skill and understanding in consistently interpreting and handling these behaviors and (2) patients' beliefs that other overt behaviors to reduce tension are not acceptable. The extent to which anger and hostility are considered acceptable depends on the magnitude and frequency of expression. If hostility, which builds up slowly, is expressed early, it will certainly be less traumatic for the patient and for team members than if it is first expressed several months after the patient has been hospitalized.

The causes of anger and hostility must be determined before considering whether any interventions are necessary. Anger is not expressed at the team member who is caring for the patient or at relatives and friends, but at what that particular person represents--life, functioning, energy--all

the things the patient is in the process of losing or has already lost.[13]
As in the case of denial, these expressions of hostility and aggression
usually serve a stabilizing, though somewhat destructive function for the
patient.

The patient in the terminal stage should be allowed to grieve. Grief,
which frequently accompanies guilt, may emerge in unreasonable, hostile
accusations towards others, or it may force the patient's anger inward. (See
Chapter 6, "Death and Dying," for detailed information on grief.)

Reinforcement and Review

3.11 Briefly summarize the guidelines which you already follow regarding what to tell the cancer patient about diagnosis:

_____

_____

_____

_____

3.12 Do most patients want to be told their diagnosis?

___yes/___no

3.13 Telling the patient his diagnosis may precipitate severe emotional problems, including death.

___true/___false

3.14 The physician's practice of revealing the diagnosis is based on:

1. _____

2. _____

3. _____

3.15 List the major characteristics of communication during the initial stage of cancer and before treatment starts:

1. _____

2. _____

3.16 During the advancing stage, difficulties in communication may be attributed to:

1. _____

2. _____

3.17 The major characteristic in the terminal stage is:

_____

3.18 The most frequently used defense mechanism of the dying patient is:

_____

3.19 The patient's hostile behavior may be primarily attributed to:

1. _____

2. _____

3.20 If you were going to intervene, list the basic precautions you would take:

1. _____

2. _____

3. _____

3.21 Should the terminal patient be allowed to grieve?

___yes/___no

Answers to Questions 3.11 3.21

3.11   Your background, training, understanding, and philosophy will influ-
       ence your selection. Basic assumptions are that (1) patients should
       not be told anything until an histological diagnosis has been estab-
       lished, (2) patients should be informed of the nature and possible
       progression of their disease, (3) all communications should be open
       and honest, and (4) patients usually have more emotional resources
       that those for which they are given credit.

3.12   Yes. Physicians differ widely in their practice of revealing the
       diagnosis, so patients may or may not be told.

3.13   False. This is a common belief, but is unfounded.

3.14   (1) belief that death is synonymous with defeat. (2) connotation
       cancer carries of death. (3) necessity of maintaining hope whenever
       possible. Hope is the central point around which the patient's
       thoughts revolve. It is consequently the critical element in the
       communication process.

3.15   (1) direct. (2) truthful.

3.16   (1) lack of desire to communicate. (2) use of defense mechanisms.

3.17   withdrawal or detachment.

3.18   denial.

3.19   (1) team members' difficulty in understanding and interpreting patient
       behavior. (2) lack of appropriate means of reducing tension.

3.20   (1) determine cause of anger and hostility. (2) determine why anger
       and hostility were directed at a particular person. (3) determine
       whether the patient's hostile behavior served any stablizing or con-
       structive function.

       If you are skilled in making interventions you know it is impossible
       to answer based on the minimal information presented. It would be
       necessary to have access to the patient's records and then to meet
       with team members and the patient before deciding on a particular
       course of action. It should be determined whether you are competent
       to make the intervention in such emotion-provoking siutations such
       as those experienced by terminally ill patients. If you are not
       skilled in making interventions, get someone who is competent to deal
       with terminally ill patients.

3.21   Yes. Grieving is obviously a way of relieving tension and is a natural
       expression. All patients will express their grief in some form during
       their illness.

Initiating Communication with Cancer Patients

Cancer patients have the same life interests, biases, and need for companionship and understanding as other persons. Some of the fears of cancer patients are: loss of independence, being left alone to die or suffer, possible disfigurement, pain, and suffocation. Communication with the cancer patient can take place on verbal and/or nonverbal levels.

Verbal communication. Some general findings on verbal communication are:

1. Most dying persons who bring up the issues of death want to talk about them.[8]

2. Many patients would be willing to talk about death if medical personnel would bring themselves to face the problem.

3. Team members can help the patient by letting him talk about cancer and death when he is ready to do so. The team member can also recognize the behavioral cues which indicate a need for a change in tactics or for an intervention. Interventions are helpful in making the patient comfortable.[9]

4. Patients should not be ignored when expressing feelings about death. Team members, by providing the patient with realistic cues or appropriate responses, can help the terminal cancer patient handle his fears until he is able to cope with them directly and face death at his own pace.

Nothing is more pathetic than the incurable patient who knows the truth about his condition, even though he has not been "officially" informed, and who desperately needs to talk to someone about his problems. He continues to act and speak as though he does not know his diagnosis and is deprived of the relief afforded by getting his feelings out in the open.[19]

Nonverbal communications. Ideally, team members would be able to recognize symptoms which are communicated at the nonverbal level. The validity of these nonverbal cues could be interpreted and evaluated along with physical symptoms. Perceptive, vigilant team members can pick up these cues and seek out contact with the patient before crisis situations develop. Recognition and accurate interpretation of nonrational subliminal emotional aspects of communication are extremely important. For example, nonverbal cues, which may be a subterfuge for anxiety, are often accompanied by complaints, constant calling for nurses, etc.[12]

In some instances nonverbal cues such as facial expressions and gestures may be readily interpreted. Nonverbal cues identified as salient for depression are eyes, mouth, and angle of head. In general, most depressed patients exhibit minimal eye contact, may have tears in their eyes, have a drawn or quivering mouth, and angle their heads downward. Ferster's[6] functional analysis of depression provides information on behavior and on environmental variables.

The following points related to nonverbal communication may be helpful in dealing with the cancer patient:

1. Touching, too infrequently done, is certainly one of the most important forms of communication with the dying person. Some persons, however, have an aversion to being touched.[8]

2. Interest, compassion, and empathy can be communicated through gestures, eye contact, and facial expressions.

3. Shared silences may be far more profound than words[8] as nonverbal communication can fill or explain silences.[4]

4. Nonverbal communications can often be effective when persons wishing to communicate are unsure of themselves, or do not know what to say

or how to say it.

5. Nonverbal communications may contradict a verbal message.

Facilitating Communications with the Cancer Patient

1. The most effective way to facilitate communication is obvious--be
    a good listener. The nondirective approach of reflecting feeling,
    restating key words, nodding your head, and other similar eliciting
    techniques which reflect your sensitivity and integrity will pro-
    vide sufficient encouragement for the patient.

2. Taking a genuine interest in the patient is an obvious way of
    starting conversations. Whether a patient communicates his fears
    and concerns will depend on trust and understanding, both of which
    build up slowly. By conveying a "caring" attitude, it should be
    possible to bridge most communication gaps.

3. By making an effort to see the illness from the patient's point
    of view, you will come to a good understanding of the patient and
    his problems. This understanding will facilitate communication.
    You must, however, be aware of your own stimulus value, i.e, how
    the other person sees you. He may consider you as a friend, as a
    confidant, or as a somewhat impersonal authority figure. His
    perceptions may or may not be accurate.

4. The best way to cheer a fatally ill person and to get him to talk
    is by giving up the notion that he needs cheering. Artificial
    cheerfulness blocks communication in the area of most concern to
    the patient--his distress and his illness.[16] Take the patient
    seriously and convey to him that he is appreciated as a person.
    If you think of yourself as a form of medication, determine an

adequate (but not toxic) dosage.[8]

Increasing Effectiveness of Communication

Methods used in communicating with cancer patients are the same as those used in daily conversation. However, in some instances, patients may be temporarily physically incapacitated or emotionally overwhelmed with their illness or treatment and appear not to hear or understand what has been said. It may be necessary to speak more slowly and distinctly (but in a normal voice) and to repeat or rephrase questions and instructions to clarify meaning. If the patient has a speech or language problem or a hearing deficit, gesturing, writing, pointing to pictures, and demonstrating may be appropriate. The patient may become very frustrated if he is not given sufficient time to make what he feels to be a satisfactory response or if he feels you have misunderstood him.

Facilitating Communication in the Health Care Team

Clarification of the roles and responsibilities of team members should break down some of the previously existing barriers to verbal communication. As team members continue to work together, their pool of shared knowledge will steadily increase. Staff conferences and scheduled and impromptu conferences with the patient, his family, and agency personnel will enhance information sharing and communication. All members of the team including the patient will benefit from free and open communication.

The patient's medical record is undoubtedly the best source of information. A detailed medical record provides a common base of knowledge as well as a vehicle for communication among team members, particularly if data are presented in a problem-oriented format.[10,20,21,22,23] The problem-oriented method consists of the application of consistent scientific methods of problem-solving to the compilation of medical records.

The problem-oriented medical record system, developed by Weed, is a logic and display system consisting of:

1. a data base, which includes the biological data obtained from the history, physical examination, and the laboratory tests.

2. an initial problem list which denotes all of the patient's problems.

3. development of plans for each problem and modification of the problem list.

4. problem-oriented recording of orders.

5. progress notes, which represent the most crucial part of the problem-oriented record, as the doctor describes the results of his actions in the following unstructured form:

    a. noting the subjective results of his work from the patient's own comments.

    b. recording any objective aspects which he notices.

    c. analyzing subjective and objective aspects.

    d. designating plans for therapy.

6. discharge notes summarizing the data base which enable the physician to arrive at his final conclusions regarding the patient.

7. audit of the medical record.

The problem-oriented system can be used to:

1. increase the effectiveness of clinical teaching, since specific areas in which the house staff needs guidance, information, or references can be readily identified.

2. improve the quality of medical care through the immediate recognition and resolution of patients' problems.

3. provide the potential for quality control of medical care since
    the problem-oriented approach is easier to audit than traditional
    record keeping techniques.

The problem-oriented record system is being taught in most medical
schools and is enthusiastically received by medical school students. It
is also very popular with residents in primary care. However, the system
is not too well accepted by the older physician. It is anticipated that
in the near future the problem-oriented approach will be in greater use at
the community hospital level and in general practice.

A problem-oriented approach to the recording of psychosocial problems
is currently being investigated.[1] Application of this method, which incor-
porates many of the procedures outlined above, will:

1. enhance the objectivity and specificity with which team members,
    allied health personnel, and students state and record psychosocial
    problems.

2. enable the psychosocial staff to spend more time treating problems
    and less time in locating and talking with staff members to clarify
    obscure, impressionistic language.

3. enable physicians to copy psychosocial information verbatim from
    medical charts for discharge summaries.

94

Reinforcement and Review

3.22 What are some basic guidelines in discussing death with a terminally
ill patient?

    1. _____

    2. _____

    3. _____

3.23 Nonverbal cues are always easy to observe and interpret.

    ___true/___false

3.24 Typical nonverbal cues for depression are:

    1. _____

    2. _____

    3. _____

    4. _____

3.25 Most effective ways of facilitating communication are:

    1. _____

    2. _____

    3. _____

    4. _____

3.26 List what you feel to be the most important aspects in increasing
communication effectiveness:

    1. _____

    2. _____

3.27 How may communication between health care team members be facilitated?

    1. _____

    (Complete your answer on the next page.)

2. _____

3. _____

Answers to Questions 3.22 - 3.27

3.22   (1) Don't bring up the topic of death or discuss death unless the
       patient indicates he is ready. (2) If the patient wants to talk
       about death, listen to him. (3) Provide emotional support or get
       support for the patient who needs emotional help.

3.23   False. Team members should receive instruction in methods used in
       recognizing and interpreting nonverbal communications, and they should
       do some research in the area. Nonverbal cues may be more important
       than verbal communication and may be unconscious manifestations of
       anxiety, hostility, and grief.

3.24   (1) decreased eye contact. (2) drawn in mouth. (3) eyes and head
       downward. (4) tears in eyes. There are many other nonverbal cues,
       although the listed ones are most common. Perceptive team and
       family members will recognize them.

3.25   (1) Be a good listener. (2) Take an interest in the patient.
       (3) Try to see the patient's point of view. (4) Take the patient
       seriously. Other ways may be equally effective, but being a good
       listener is extremely important. A nondirective approach is often
       most effective.

3.26   Being patient and understanding are both important, but there is no
       specific answer to this question. Methods you have used in the past
       to increase effectiveness of communication should be appropriate.

3.27   (1) clarify roles and responsibilities. (2) establish open channels
       of communication between team members. (3) share knowledge.

FACTORS INFLUENCING THE COMMUNICATION PROCESS

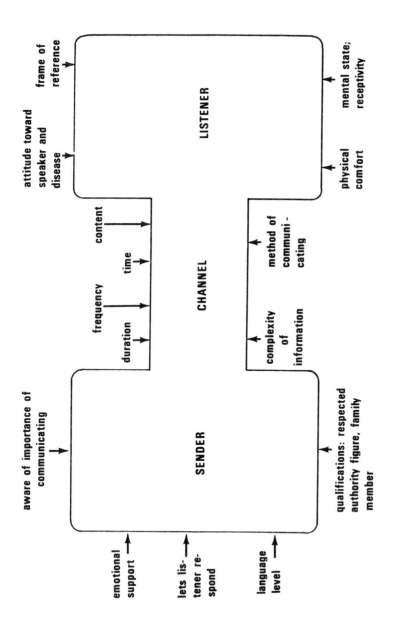

References

1. Abrams, K.S., Neville, R., & Becker, M.C. Problem-oriented recording of psychosocial problems. Arch. Phys. Med. Rehabil., 1973, 54, 316-319.

2. Abrams, R.D. The patient with cancer--his changing pattern of communication. New England Journal of Medicine, 1966, 274 (6), 317-322.

3. Branch, C.H.H. Psychiatric aspects of malignant disease. CA, Bull. Can. Prog., 1956, 6, 102-104.

4. Coleman, J.C., & Hammen, C.L. Contemporary psychology and effective behavior. Glenview, Ill.: Scott, Foresman and Co., 1974.

5. Feder, S.L. Psychological considerations in the care of patients with cancer. Ann. N.Y. Acad. Sci., 1966, 125, 1020-1027.

6. Ferster, C.B. A functional analysis of depression. Am. Psychol., 1973, 28, 857-870.

7. Ford, C.S. Ego-adaptive mechanisms of older persons. Social Casework, 1965, 46, 16-21.

8. Grollman, E.A. (Ed.). Concerning death: a practical guide for the living. Boston: Beacon Press, 1974.

9. Heusinkveld, K.B. Cues to communication with the terminal cancer patient. Nursing Forum, 1972, 11, 105-113.

10. Hurst, J.W., Walker, H.K. (Eds.). The problem-oriented system. New York: Medcom Press, 1972.

11. Kelly, W.D., & Friesen, S.R. Do cancer patients want to be told? Surgery, 1950, 27, 822-826.

12. Klagsbrun, S.C. Cancer, nurses, and emotions. RN, 1970, 33 (1), 46-51.

13. Kubler-Ross, E. What is it like to be dying? Am. J. Nursing, 1971, 71 (1), 54-60.

14. Munn, N.L. Psychology (5th ed.). New York: Houghton Mifflin Co., 1961.

15. Oken, D. What to tell cancer patients: a study of medical attitudes. J.A.M.A., 1961, 175, 1120-1128.

16. Payne, E.C., & Krant, M.D. The psychosocial aspects of advanced cancer. J.A.M.A., 1969, 210, 1238-1242.

17. Samp, R.J., & Curreri, A.R. Questionnaire survey on public cancer education obtained from cancer patients and their families. Cancer, 1957, 10, 382-384.

18. Shands, H.C., Finesinger, J.E., Cobb, S., Abrams, R.D. Psychological mechanisms in patients with cancer. Cancer, 1951, 4, 1159-1170.

19. Stehlin, J.S., Jr., & Beach, K.H. Psychological aspects of cancer therapy. J.A.M.A., 1966, 197, 100.

20. Weed, L.L. Medical records, medical education, and patient care. Cleveland: The Press of Case Western Reserve University, 1969.

21. Weed, L.L. Medical records that guide and teach. New England J. Med., 1968, 278, 593-600; 652-657.

22. Weed, L.L. Quality control and the medical record. Arch. Intern. Med., 1971, 127, 101-105.

23. Weed, L.L. Technology is a link, not a barrier, for doctor and patient. Modern Hospital, 1970, 114, 80-83.

Suggested Readings

Hall, C.S., Lindzey, G. Theories of personality (2nd ed.). New York: John Wiley & Sons, 1970.

Krant, M.J. Dying and dignity: the meaning and control of a personal death. Springfield, Ill.: Charles C Thomas, 1974.

Kubler-Ross, E. On death and dying. New York: The Macmillan Co., 1969.

Smith, E.A., & Taylor, G.H. Increasing listening effectiveness. Texas Medicine, 1975, 70 (9), 80-83.

Weisman, A.D. Dying and denying. New York: Behavioral Books, 1972.

Chapter 4

PERSONALITY AND ADJUSTMENT

Personality research has revealed that at one time or another all persons experience stressful situations, some of which may be life-threatening. Responses to these stressful situations are greatly influenced by the individual's personality, his adjustment to his environment,and to the magnitude and duration of the stress producing situation.

The distinguishing characteristics of cancer patients are (1) their frequent interpretation of the diagnosis of cancer as being synonymous with death and (2) their typical reactions to this life-threatening diagnosis. As presented in Chapter 2, the responses made by cancer patients differ from those made by the "average" person in (1) frequency, (2) intensity, (3) duration of response, and (4) resultant personal ineffectiveness. When the expression of these responses or behaviors is consistently inappropriate or deviates from some expected, realistic standard of behavior, all persons, including the cancer patient, require the assistance of team members who are skilled in making interventions.

This chapter includes sections on (1) personality, (2) individual differences, (3) self-image, and (4) feeling and emotion. The information presented will provide an overview of personality and adjustment and should facilitate the understanding of behavior in general.

Personality

Personality consists of a set of descriptive terms or values which are used to describe a person being studied according to certain variables or dimensions occupying a central position within the particular theory utilized.[5]

Personality may be defined as the dynamic organization within the individual of those perceptual, cognitive, emotional, and motivational systems which determine his unique response to his environment.[8] Further analysis of Stagner's comprehensive definition of personality includes the following:

1. perceptual--related to the senses such as audition, sight, touch, and smell. Perceptual style is the process of perceiving; it involves a constant interaction of present stimulation and past experience.

2. cognitive--memory and reasoning.

3. emotional--anxiety, depression, fear, and other affective reactions.

4. motivational--the inner control of behavior as represented by physiological conditions, interests, attitudes, and aspirations.[6]

5. unique--individual, or possessed by only one person.

6. response--way of reacting to a stimulus which may be usual ("normal" or expected) or unusual ("abnormal"* or unexpected).

The concept of homeostasis permeates the study of personality. The restoration of steady temperature by the body and the maintenance of carbon dioxide in the blood stream are examples of physiological homeostasis. Personality may be a pattern of steady states valued by the person. These states are expressions of unique personality characteristics. Personality may also be conceptualized from a hedonistic, psychoanalytical, cognitive, or behavioristic standpoint. The text by Hall and Lindzey[5] is an excellent

---

*Psychologists refrain from designating certain behaviors (responses) "normal" or "abnormal," as each behavior must be analyzed in terms of the person's traits, predispositions, the immediate situation which prompted the response, and the stresses which the person is experiencing.

source of information on personality theory.

Individual Differences

Another common approach to the study of personality is through individual differences.[10] Personality may be meaningfully analyzed according to the unique pattern of surface and source traits*. Individual differences in traits may be investigated, but such investigations are complex and time-consuming. The difficulty in studying traits may be attributed to the fact that approximately 18,000 personality trait names have been identified.[1] Factor analytic studies and other methods of investigation have revealed that many of the names assigned to traits are similar.

The major factors contributing to individual differences are heredity, environment, maturation, and learning. The most important ways in which individuals differ are[9]:

1. physical size

2. sex

3. age

4. intelligence

5. aptitude

6. personality

7. interests

---

*Trait: that which is inferred from actual observations of behavior. There are thousands of surface traits, many of which may be grouped together. Surface traits are observable, relatively stable behaviors which appear in interpersonal contacts or responses to stimuli, e.g., cheerfulness, liveliness, etc. Source traits underlie structures which are not expressed directly, but are expressed through the medium of surface traits. Examples of source traits are honesty, resourcefulness, stability, etc.

8. attitudes

9. perception[6]

    a. vision

    b. hearing

    c. smell

    d. touch

    e. taste

    f. equilibrium

    g. <u>kinesthesis</u>

10. feeling and emotion

11. race and nationality

12. socioeconomic level

    Individual differences is the approach to personality that seems most appropriate for the study of cancer patients. Characteristics that most frequently differentiate cancer patients from other patients or persons are those which relate to feeling and emotion and to perception. The cancer patient's perception and interpretation of what is going on around him may be permanently or temporarily clouded by his use of such ego defense mechanisms as repression and denial.

Reinforcement and Review

4.1 Check the words that are included in Stagner's definition of person-
     ality:

    1. __perception   8. __intellectual
    2. __cognition   9. __individual dif-
    3. __constant   ferences
    4. __emotional or affective   10. __dynamic
        aspects   11. __expectancy
    5. __motivation   12. __abnormal
    6. __uniqueness of response 13. __well adjusted
    7. __environment   14. __physical

4.2 (1) Draw a small circle in the middle of the rectangle presented below.
     (2) Draw four arrows pointing <u>out</u> from the circle and four arrows
         pointing <u>toward</u> the circle.
     (3) Label the inward pointing arrows with the forces, elements, or
         daily activities influencing the cancer patient. These forces
         can be based on material presented in chapters 2 and 3 in this
         text or on your own experience.
     (4) Label the outward pointing arrows with the four personality factors
         which influence the patient to react in specific ways. Your dia-
         gram will be a pictorial representation of the environment, as
         represented by the rectangle, the forces acting on the patient,
         and his typical or expected responses. You may think of many more
         factors than those listed.

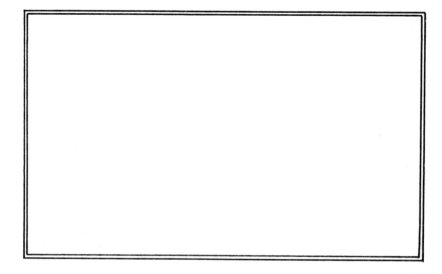

4.3 The study of personality may be approached from which perspectives or theories?

      1. _____   4. _____

      2. _____   5. _____

      3. _____   6. _____

4.4 Which theory or approach to the study of personality is most appropriate for the study of the cancer patient?

      _____

4.5 How are surface traits and source traits differentiated?

      _____

      _____

4.6 Are surface and source traits easy to differentiate?

      ___yes/___no. Why? _____

      _____

4.7 (1) Draw a circle with an approximate diameter of 3 inches.
    (2) Draw another circle with an approximate diameter of 2 inches within the larger circle. These concentric circles represent your personality.
    (3) Think of your own most common and predominating personality characteristics. You may wish to include personality traits attributed to you by others.
    (4) Determine which of these personality traits are surface traits and which are source traits.
    (5) Write the names of each of the surface traits on the outside of the larger circle or in the space between the two circles. Write the names of each of the source-traits inside the inner circle.

    Use the next page to draw your diagram.

4.8 List five major ways in which individuals (not necessarily cancer
     patients) differ:

    1. _____   4. _____

    2. _____   5. _____

    3. _____

4.9 With respect to individual differences, what characteristics distinguish
     cancer patients from other persons?

    _____

    _____

Answers to Questions 4.1 - 4.9

4.1   1, 2, 4, 5, 6, 7, 10, 11

4.2   Inward pointing arrows representing daily activities influencing the
cancer patient might include: treatment procedures, cost of treatment,
interactions with team members, physical limitations of the environment,
needs of family.

Outward pointing arrows representing personality factors influencing the
patient to react in specific ways might include: anxiety, guilt, withdrawal, fear, hostility, desire for social acceptance, desire to be
productive, etc.

4.3   homeostatic, behavioristic, individualistic, psychoanalytic, cognitive,
hedonistic, and other approaches with which you are familiar.

4.4   Homeostasis or maintenance of equilibrium is a logical first choice.
From a broad perspective, homeostasis implies maintenance of both
physical and mental equilibrium. However, since emotional disturbances
and mental illness occur in approximately 20%[3] of the general population,
about the same percentage of cancer patients may be emotionally or
mentally disturbed. Also, the person who has been diagnosed as having
cancer faces a stress situation which may precipitate an emotional
crisis that would not have occurred normally. No specific evidence
exists to document or disclaim this thought, however.

4.5   Surface traits are observable, and source traits are inferred from
behavior.

4.6   No, because (1) there are so many traits and (2) trait names are similar.

4.7   Most persons experience difficulty in determining their own enduring
personality characteristics. The task of differentiating surface and
source traits is not easy. However, this exercise has provided information about yourself that may be helpful in your interpersonal
relationships.

4.8   physical size, age, sex, aptitude, personality, interests, intelligence,
attitudes, perception, feeling and emotion. Race, nationality, and
socioeconomic level also influence personality and behavior.

4.9   There are no specific distinguishing characteristics. However,
perception may be less acute, and feeling and emotion flattened in
affect. The cancer patient's typical modes of reacting are adversely
influenced by his preoccupation with his disease.

Self-Image

The self is the central nucleus around which the personality develops.[8] In temporal terms, the self is the point between the present and the future. The self includes conscious and unconscious components. Man continually strives to maintain and enhance his perceived self.[4]

The self-image is the image a person carries around with him of his own attributes including emotions, motivations, and beliefs. The self-image is the earliest form of body image. It includes an evaluation of oneself which is largely obtained from the individual's own observations and from the evaluations of others. This feedback provides the person with information about his attitudes, beliefs, values, and behavior. Since the self-image is segmented, a person may perceive himself differently at different times.

A person's perception of his body image is of great importance; he may hear himself described as strong, active, or nervous, for example, and these descriptions may reinforce or oppose his conception of himself.

The self-image of a cancer patient is particularly vulnerable, especially in instances where there are physical changes, such as those that result from facial surgery or amputation. The significance of the body part or body area affected by cancer must be considered from the standpoint of how the loss or disfigurement affects (1) vital body function, (2) psychological adjustment, (3) social adjustment, (4) occupational and vocational status. These matters are of great concern in the rehabilitation process and are presented in more detail in Smith[7].

Since the cancer patient's ability to reason and react in a logical manner may be temporarily impaired, his perceptions of his self-image may not always be accurate. If perceptions are not accurate, it would be

advisable to help the patient develop a more positive self-image. The following suggestions may be useful:

1. If there are no obvious physical reasons such as disfigurement and
   no major adjustment problems or recently experienced emotional crises,
   try to find out what is causing the patient's negative self-image.
   If you cannot determine his problem through casual or specific
   questions, ask for help from other team members who work with the
   patient. They may provide meaningful information based on their
   personal contact or on their observations. You should also examine
   the medical record and consult with family and friends if you feel
   such consultations would be appropriate and beneficial.

2. If methods suggested above are not successful, you may find that
   the patient will be more willing to talk about himself if you express
   genuine interest and concern.

3. If you are still dissatisfied with the results, other team members
   trained in counseling and interview techniques may assist you. This
   assistance may consist of an interview by a clinical psychologist
   or the administration of psychological tests such as personality
   measures. One commonly used and well accepted technique which may
   be used or specifically developed for use is the Q-sort. This
   technique allows for the classification of descriptive statements
   about the patient's personality into "self" and "ideal self" categories; categories range from "most like me" to "least like me."
   The scoring and interpretation of this test does require some
   knowledge of psychological testing procedures. The Q-sort is more
   likely to be used in clinical assessment than in daily hospital

routine. Clinical and social psychologists are quite familiar with Q-sort techniques. Many other methods of obtaining information regarding the patient's personality and adjustment may be used, however.

Feeling and Emotion

Emotion may be defined as an aroused desire. It also may be considered as an activated or excited state that underlies the experiences and actions which occur in fear, rage, sorrow, delight, horror, grief, love, and other emotional states. In its most obvious manifestations, emotion is an acute condition characterized by disruption of everyday experiences and activities.[6]

The most common expressions of feeling and emotions are:

1. verbal--crying, laughing, screaming.

2. nonverbal--body movements, gestures, grimaces, smiles, postures.

3. physiological--production of adrenalin and noradrenalin by the adrenal gland, increased heart rate, secretion of steroids in the urine, sweaty palms, etc.

Anxiety is an emotional state in which there is a vague, generalized feeling of fear. It may also be defined as a state of emotional tension characterized by apprehension and fearfulness. Anxiety is likely to be diffuse, while fear is frequently tied to a specific stimulus.[2] Anxiety may be decreased through any number of commonly accepted methods such as psychotherapy, relaxation techniques, and oral medication such as Valium and Dalmane.

Individual differences exist in generalized anxiety with respect to:

1. emotional responsiveness--This involves the magnitude of responses to a given intensity of stimulation.

2. nonverbal measure of anxiety--This includes voice pitch, body

movements, gestures, facial expressions, and other expressive traits. Indications of anxiety may be reflected in at least ten measures of physiological activity. Changes in palmar sweating, heart rate, blood pressure, steadiness, and <u>EEGs</u>, for instance, may be signals of anxiety.

3. psychiatric symptoms--Although anxiety may be a factor in certain psychotic and neurotic behaviors, personality and environmental variables play significant roles.

Although all persons experience feelings of anxiety at one time or another, the intensity of the anxiety is much greater in cancer patients. Cancer patients may also experience anxiety for prolonged periods of time. Anxiety may produce devastating effects on cancer patients.

Emotions may serve as helpers (adaptive) or as hinderers (disruptive). In mild emotion there is a slight increase in tension which usually improves performance on most tasks.

Reinforcement and Review

4.10 How would you begin to help a patient to develop a more positive self-image?

    1. _____

    2. _____

    3. _____

4.11 Define emotion:

    _____

    _____

4.12 Define anxiety:

    _____

4.13 Using your own words, list the emotions cancer patients experience:

    _____

    _____

4.14 What are some ways of decreasing anxiety?

    _____

    _____

4.15 What are the major individual differences in generalized anxiety?

    1. _____

    2. _____

    3. _____

4.16 In what two major ways do emotions function?

    _____ and _____

Answers to Questions 4.10 - 4.16

4.10 (1) Determine the cause of the negative self-image by talking to the patient and consulting family and other team members. (2) Express genuine interest and concern to draw the patient out. (3) Use counseling, interview, and particular skills of other team members.

4.11 an aroused desire, an activated or excited state. Many other synonyms or definitions are acceptable.

4.12 an emotional state in which there is a vague, generalized feeling of fear.

4.13 The emotions listed should have been based on the material presented in chapters 2 and 3. Typical emotions are fear, anxiety, insecurity, and depression. Although the emotions you listed frequently occur in other persons, they occur with greater frequency and intensity and last longer in cancer patients than they do in other persons. If you wish, you may refer back to the first page of this chapter.

4.14 psychotherapy, relaxation techniques, and oral medication (tranquilizers).

4.15 (1) increased emotional responsiveness. (2) increased anxiety as expressed by nonverbal measures. (3) appearance of psychiatric symptoms (psychotic and neurotic behaviors).

4.16 helpers (adaptive) and hinderers (disruptive).

Definitions

1. adrenal gland--an endocrine gland which secretes adrenalin and noradrenalin.

2. adrenalin--the trade name for epinephrine, a hormone produced by the supra-renal glands. It acts to constrict blood vessels, control bleeding, and raise blood pressure.

3. EEG (electroencephalogram)--a record of electrical rhythms associated with some brain activities. EEG's are recorded with an electroencephalo-graph.

4. homeostasis--the organism takes action to protect or to restore certain favorable steady states.

5. kinesthesis--muscle and movement sense mediated by the receptors in the muscles, tendons, and joints.

6. noradrenalin--a secretion of the adrenal medulla (along with adrenalin) and also of nerve-endings in the sympathetic nervous system.

7. steroids--a group name for compounds that resemble cholesterol chemically and include such substances as sex hormones, bile acids, sterols proper and some of the cancerogenic hydrocarbons.

References

1. Allport, G.W., & Odbert, A.A. Trait names, a psycholexical study. Psychol. Monogr., 1936, 47, 1-171.

2. Byrne, D. An introduction to personality (2nd ed.). New Jersey: Prentice-Hall, 1974.

3. Coleman, J.C. Abnormal psychology and modern life (3rd ed.). Chicago: Scott, Foresman and Co., 1964.

4. Combs, A.W., & Snygg, D. Individual behavior (Rev. ed.). New York: Harper, 1959.

5. Hall, C.S., & Lindzey, G. Theories of personality (2nd ed.). New York: John Wiley & Sons, 1970.

6. Munn, N.L. Psychology (5th ed.). New York: Houghton Mifflin Co., 1961.

7. Smith, E.A. A comprehensive approach to rehabilitation of the cancer patient. (A publication of The University of Texas Health Science Center at Houston, Division of Continuing Education, 1975.)

8. Stagner, R. Psychology of personality (4th ed.). New York: McGraw-Hill, 1974.

9. Tyler, L.E. The psychology of human differences (2nd ed.). New York: Appleton-Century-Crofts, Inc., 1956.

10. Underwood, B.J. Individual differences as a crucible in theory construction. Amer. Psychol., 1975, 30, 128-134.

Chapter 5

PAIN

A common belief supported by the public and by many health care professionals is that cancer patients always experience pain.[4] On the contrary, it
is the absence of pain that frequently keeps persons who have potentially
cancerous swellings or other unexplainable signs or symptoms from going to
their physician. Twycross reports that as many as 50% of all cancer patients
experience no pain or have minimal discomfort, 40% have severe pain, and 10%
have less intense pain.[15] In general, pain occurs when the tumor causes obstruction, initiates infection, or involves nerves.[1] Pain may be a serious problem in certain types of cancer and cause an extremely difficult problem in
clinical management.

There is no completely satisfactory definition of pain. Pain may be
defined medically as "a more or less localized sensation of discomfort, distress, or agony, resulting from the stimulation of specialized nerve end-
ings."[8] Pain may be considered to be: (1) a response to noxious stimulation,
(2) an experience that is both perception and reaction,[4] (3) a signal of biological malfunction, and (4) a message to the ego to take evasive action
to protect the integrity of the body.[14]

One of the main problems in systematically investigating and accurately
reporting on pain perception is that the majority of research relies on
introspective reports. Few reported studies deal with pain on a day-to-day
basis.

Although pain is commonly dichotomized into organic and psychogenic
categories, these convenient clinical classifications often lead to errors

in patient management. The errors may be attributed to the difficulty in clearly delineating the cause of pain.

Causes of Organic Pain

Some factors which produce pain in cancer are: (1) compression of spinal sensory nerve roots, trunks, or nerve plexuses by a tumor mass, (2) infiltration of the nerves and the blood vessels by tumor cells, (3) distention or obstruction of a hollow viscus or of a solid organ due to obstruction by tumor, (4) obstruction of blood vessel by tumor which causes ischemia of distal tissues and nerves, (5) necrosis, infection, and inflammation of tissue adjacent to the tumor, and (6) pathological fracture of the bone in the metastatic disease; the bone becomes very fragile and breaks spontaneously.[5]

Pathological conditions such as loss of fluid and electrolytes in the body fluids or drainage, depression, anorexia, nausea and vomiting, and diarrhea are major threats to the patient's nutritional status. Patients who do not receive adequate nutrition become weak, debilitated, physically immobile, increasingly depressed, worried, and anxious. These patients obviously experience more discomfort and pain than those who are well nourished.[4]

Factors Related to Psychogenic Pain

Pain produces emotional changes in well adjusted persons. Dependency needs, self-centeredness, and secondary gain are increased. Culture influences the patient's interpretation of pain, as well as his feelings about what should be done about pain. Some cultures accept pain as part of the human condition, but in the United States, considerable effort is directed toward avoiding, controlling, or eliminating pain.[4]

Environmental factors also play a role. For instance, pain tends to be worse at nights because the patient is more aware of himself; he has more time to worry, think about his future, his family, and other personal and physical problems. The patient may experience anxiety and pain at night because he feels alone, yet he may forget his pain during daytime recreational activities.[13]

Guilt frequently accompanies pain. Many cancer patients experience feelings of guilt as they search for some meaning in the stressful experiences they suffer. They may have unresolved feelings of ill will and hostility toward others or feel that they are being punished for something they did in the past.[4]

Intensity of Pain

The intensity of the experience of pain is influenced by: (1) the unique past history and personality of the patient, (2) the meaning the patient gives to the pain producing situation, and (3) the patient's present "state of mind."[12] Consequently, pain may be a function of the individual.

There is no consistent, direct relationship between size of wound and pain intensity.[4] Persons whose malignancies and surgical procedures were similar often experience great differences in postoperative pain.

Separating physical pain from fear of pain and painful anxieties is difficult. Anxiety, which is frequently experienced by cancer patients, intensifies pain.[6] Anxiety also appears to be a factor in determining an individual's ability to tolerate or endure pain.[4]

Individual Differences

Psychophysical research has demonstrated inter-individual and intra-individual differences in pain thresholds.[2] In addition to perceptual differences, persons vary in accuracy when estimating the magnitude of pain. At one end of the continuum are "augmenters," who consistently increase the magnitude of sensory data and tolerate pain for short periods. At the other end of the continuum are "reducers," who consistently decrease the magnitude of sensory data and tolerate pain for long periods.[4]

Pain Thresholds

Verbal instructions (hypnosis), biofeedback, analgesics, and other stimuli readily influence pain thresholds. Attention and anticipation raise the patient's anxiety, which then increases the intensity of the perceived pain.[12]

Figure 1 outlines the source, meaning, and interpretation of pain[14]:

SOURCE OF PAIN	MEANING	INTERPRETATION
body involved	medical meaning	a signal of biological malfunction
body and other people	communicative meaning	as a fundamental method of asking for help or attention
some particular person	knowing to whom the pain communication is being addressed	may signify rejection, aggression or a myriad of other interpersonal communications

Fig. 1 Source, Meaning, and Interpretation of Pain

Reinforcement and Review

5.1 Define pain in your own words:

_____

5.2 How is pain classified clinically?

_____ and _____

5.3 Why is the classification of pain into organic and psychogenic categories
     inappropriate?

_____

5.4 What is the most frequent focus of research on pain?

_____

5.5 What is introspective report?

_____

5.6 What are three causes of organic pain?

     1. _____

     2. _____

     3. _____

5.7 The intensity of pain is influenced by:

     1. _____

     2. _____

     3. _____

5.8 Recall an experience in which you experienced pain. Write down your
     emotional and physical experiences:

     (Use the next page to answer the question.)

Emotional	Physical
_____	_____
_____	_____
_____	_____

5.9 Did you feel that pain actually increased at night?

   ___yes/___no (If you answered "no," go to question 5.12.)

5.10 Did pain really increase at night?

   ___yes/___no

5.11 Why did pain appear to increase at night?

   _____

5.12 List the emotional changes that pain may produce in well adjusted persons:

   1. _____

   2. _____

   3. _____

5.13 What medical and psychological procedures can be used to influence pain thresholds?

Medical	Psychological
_____	_____
_____	_____
_____	_____

5.14 After studying Fig. 1, what basic conclusions could be made about each of the following: (1) source of pain, (2) meaning of pain, (3) interpretation of pain?

   (Use the next page to answer the question.)

1. Source of pain: _____

_____

2. Meaning of pain: _____

_____

3. Interpretation of pain: _____

_____

5.15 List the sequence of steps usually taken when attempting to control the cancer patient's pain:

1. _____

2. _____

3. _____

Answers to Questions 5.1 - 5.15

5.1   Discomfort, distress, sensation of hurting, suffering are all good definitions.

5.2   organic and psychogenic (or emotional or psychological).

5.3   because of possible errors in patient management since the cause of pain is difficult to identify.

5.4   introspective report.

5.5   report based on your own personal experiences without reference to quantification or any other experimental or carefully controlled method of investigation.

5.6   any of the following: (1) compression of spinal nerves by a tumor mass. (2) infiltration of nerves and blood vessels by tumor cells. (3) distention of hollow viscus. (4) obstruction of blood vessels by tumor. (5) necrosis, infection, and inflammation of adjacent tissue to tumor. (6) pathological fracture of bone.

5.7   (1) patient's past history. (2) meaning pain has for the patient. (3) patient's present state of mind.

5.8   no specific answer. Your responses are somewhat unique, although they will be similar in a general way to experiences of cancer patients.

5.9   You probably thought it did.

5.10 From a physiological standpoint, pain probably remained constant. However, the mind has a great influence over many of our perceptions, not just pain. You may have experienced more severe pain at night.

5.11 because there was time to think and/or worry about yourself. Decreased outside stimulation such as visitors and telephone calls, the temporary halt of constructive distractions by team members as they tended to your needs, and the feelings of semi-isolation brought about by darkness make pain appear to increase at night.

5.12 (1) dependency needs increase. (2) self-centeredness increases. (3) secondary gain increases.

5.13 Medical: analgesics, pain killers, biofeedback.
      Psychological: hypnosis, biofeedback, trying to take person's mind off his pain.

5.14 (1) Source of pain: The body and the patient's interpretation (mind) may be involved, as pain can have psychological (psychogenic) sources. (2) Meaning of pain: Other than signalling biologic malfunction, pain has no meaning for the patient unless it can be directed toward a person: the surgeon who performed the pain producing operation, family members who suggested the patient come for a checkup that resulted in a painful examination or surgical procedure or other similar pain producing circumstances.

5.15 (1) Make an effort to understand the patient and deal with his fears and anxieties. (2) Try to clear up misconceptions regarding treatment and other related factors. (3) If you are a physician, you will develop the patient's treatment plan, focusing on the pain causing lesion. The nonphysician team members will report physical changes and accompanying psychological data to the physician-in-charge or team coordinator.

Differentiating between meaning and interpretation is difficult. Pain has either conscious or unconscious meaning for the patient. It is the patient's individualistic expression of his pain that can be interpreted. Do you remember the last occasion in which you exaggerated the amount of pain you experienced so you could get more attention? Don't worry, we all do this.

Treatment of Pain

The first steps in relief from cancer pain may involve working with a specialist or with members of a multi-disciplinary team who function in a "Pain Clinic." According to Chiu,[5] many hospitals are using a multidisciplinary approach to alleviate chronic, intractable pain. Members of the "Pain Clinic"* coordinate "input tactics" (physical, chemical, behavioral, or subjective techniques) and "output tactics" (retrain the central nervous system's response to painful stimuli rather than to alter its physical structure).

When medical expertise such as that described in the pain clinic is unavailable, other realistic approaches are possible. In any case, members of the team need to develop an understanding of the patient's emotional makeup and must be able to deal with his fears, anxieties, and possible misconceptions. The physician must learn the meaning of words the patient uses to describe pain and other symptoms.[11] What the patient describes as dizziness, for example, may mean lightheadedness, unsteadiness of gait, or true vertigo.

In most instances, the physical source of pain is obvious, as in surgery. The best method(s) of treating pain should be outlined in the treatment plan developed by the surgeon and appropriate team members. Any treatment for pain and discomfort should follow an orderly progression. Typical steps outlined by Hall[11] and Derrick[7] consist of (1) reviewing the patient's entire situation to find out what his disease actually is, (2) determining

---

* generalists, neurologists, neurosurgeons, orthopedic surgeons, anesthesiologists, psychiatrists, psychologists, clinical pharmacologists, physical and occupational therapists, nurses, and social workers.

the stage of the disease, (3) locating the pain so that the exact cause can be determined, and (4) controlling the regional and generalized pain.

It is important to remember that not all of the cancer patient's symptoms are caused by cancer and that the pain of cancer is often not associated with the disease as much as with a nursing problem--a painful position, dry mouth, bed sores, or cracked lips. The nurse's attitude in relieving pain is significant; severe discomfort can be greatly reduced with good nursing. Just sitting with a patient who is in pain may be helpful in terms of pain control.[3]

The common methods of treating mild pain in cancer patients include analgesics, narcotics, and tranquilizers. Each of these treatments may produce side-effects such as vertigo, headache, nausea, mental confusion, and vomiting, all of which cause discomfort and may be dangerous. The use of narcotics in pain control seldom causes any addiction problems.

For more severe or protracted pain in localized areas, the peripheral nerve block may be useful. Drugs such as xylocaine or neurolytic drugs such as absolute alcohol or phenol may provide palliation for periods up to six months. The subarachnoid block is reported to be extremely effective in treating patients with advanced cancer. However, undesirable side-effects such as necrosis, sloughing of superficial tissues, and peripheral neuritis of the blocked nerve may result.[7]

Other techniques used in pain relief include surgery, neurosurgery, precutaneous cordotomy, dorsal rhizotomy, intrathecal radiotherapy, and electrical stimulation. Intrathecal superchilled saline solution is used when neurosurgery is contraindicated or when narcotics are not beneficial because of addiction or are ineffective in dealing with pain.[7]

Physical therapy techniques including heat and cold, exercise, postural correction, traction, manipulation, massage, and hydrotherapy may be beneficial. Acupuncture, biofeedback, and hypnosis are of little value in pain control.

Chronic pain is: (1) pain that is disproportionate to the physical illness, (2) pain that apparently is not related to the underlying somatic pathology, (3) pain that does not respond to the appropriate medical treatment, or (4) any combination of the above categories.[13] Chronic pain may be experienced for varying periods of time, but is frequently considered to last a long time.

Medical treatments related to biological functioning have been notoriously erratic in the ameliorization of chronic pain.[2] The patient suffering from chronic or intractable pain is a medical problem because his pain may have emotional parameters. The physician must assume that the pain is real, however, and treat the patient accordingly.

Because of its detrimental effect on motivation, chronic pain may retard rehabilitation. Pain further impedes rehabilitation by partially or completely immobilizing the patient, causing fatigue, and producing such problems as withdrawal from activities.

Use of analgesics for temporary palliation of pain is desirable and may eliminate the need for more complicated, expensive, or morbidity-inducing therapy. The choice of the analgesic agent should be based on: (1) ease of administration, (2) cost, (3) freedom from side-effects, (4) progressive analgesia, and (5) relative effects on pain perception and tolerance.[11] These considerations as well as any possible ramifications should be discussed with the patient and, in some instances, with his family.

Phantom pain (phantom limb) and phantom sensation may occur following amputation. The patient who suffers from phantom pain complains of chronic twisting, tearing, pulling, and annoying pain. Szasz[14] and Fischer[9] report that the symptom of pain appears to be the result of an adaptive mechanism that goes awry. Patients with chronic, severe phantom pain present a clinical picture similar to the paranoid. According to Grzesiak,[10] phantom sensations result from: (1) various sources of irritation in the stump such as scar tissue, (2) neuroma, (3) lack of oxygen, and (4) nerve destruction.

Reinforcement and Review

5.16 Who manages chronic pain in many hospitals?

_____

5.17 Name as many members of the multidisciplinary team as possible:

_____

_____

_____

5.18 Are you a member of this team?

___yes/___no

5.19 If you have had surgery and suffered pain, what effective methods were used in controlling your pain?

_____

_____

5.20 Common methods of treating pain in cancer patients are:

1. _____

2. _____

3. _____

5.21 Why is chronic pain a problem?

1. _____

2. _____

3. _____

4. _____

5.22 Why are analgesics used for temporary palliation from pain?

(Use the next page to answer the question)

_____

5.23 The choice of analgesic agents is based on what main factors?

1. _____

2. _____

3. _____

4. _____

5. _____

5.24 Is phantom pain real?

___yes/___no

5.25 Phantom pain may be attributed to:

1. _____

2. _____

3. _____

4. _____

Answers to Questions 5.16 - 5.25

5.16 the multidisciplinary team.

5.17 generalists, neurologists, neurosurgeons, orthopedic surgeons, anesthesiologists, psychiatrists, psychologists, clinical pharmacologists, physical and occupational therapists, nurses, and social workers.

5.18 No answer is provided.

5.19 If your surgery was major, a spinal nerve block was probably used. In minor surgery, a common procedure is use of local anesthetics.

5.20 (1) analgesics. (2) narcotics. (3) tranquilizers.

5.21 (1) unrelated to underlying somatic pathology. (2) does not respond to appropriate medical treatment. (3) may involve emotional parameters. (4) decreases motivation and retards rehabilitation.

5.22 to eliminate the need for more complicated, expensive or morbidity-inducing therapy.

5.23 (1) ease of administration. (2) cost. (3) freedom from side-effects. (4) progressive analgesia (to be used to control pain). (5) relative effects on pain perception and tolerance.

5.24 Yes. Patients may complain that pain sensations appear to be coming from the part of the limb that has been amputated. If patients experience prolonged phantom pain (3 months or more), some thought should be given to enlisting the assistance of a clinical psychologist or psychiatrist who could determine whether the patient has severe emotional or mild paranoid tendencies.

5.25 (1) irritation in the stump. (2) neuroma. (3) lack of oxygen. (4) nerve destruction.

Definitions

1. analgesic--(1) relieving pain, (2) not sensitive as to pain, (3) an agent
    that alleviates pain without causing loss of consciousness (aspirin, Darvon).

2. ischemia--deficiency of blood in a part, due to functional construction
    or actual obstruction of a blood vessel.

3. narcotic--(1) pertaining to or producing narcosis, (2) an agent that
    produces insensibility or stupor.

4. necrosis--death of tissue, usually as individual cells, groups of cells,
    or in small localized areas.

5. neuroma--small bulb-like growth of nerve fibers and connective tissue;
    may be extremely sensitive and painful.

6. organic--(1) pertaining to an organ or the organs, (2) having an organized
    structure, (3) arising from an organism, (4) pertaining to substances
    derived from living organisms.

7. palliative--(1) affording relief but not cure, (2) an alleviating medicine.

8. paranoid--disorder characterized by transient, poorly systematized delu-
    sions of persecution and/or grandeur.

9. pathologic--indicative of or caused by a morbid condition.

10. plexus--a netwerk or tangle; used in anatomical nomenclature as a general
    term to designate a network of lymphatic vessels, nerves, or veins.

11. viscus--any large interior organ in any one of the three great cavities
    of the body, especially in the abdomen.

References

1. American Cancer Society. A cancer source book for nurses. American Cancer Society, Inc., 1975.

2. Barber, T.X. Toward a theory of pain: relief of chronic pain by prefrontal leucotomy, opiates, placebos, and hypnosis. Psychological Bulletin, 1969, 56, 430-460.

3. Barckley, V. Enough time for good nursing. Nursing Outlook, 1964, 12, (4), 44-48.

4. Benoliel, J.Q., & Crowley, D.M. The patient in pain: new concepts. In Proceedings of the national conference on cancer nursing. New York: American Cancer Society, Inc., 1974.

5. Chiu, W.J. Based on notes used by Dr. Chiu in his presentation on "Pain" for the "Continuing Education Program for Physical and Occupational Therapists," October 24, 1974.

6. Cobb, A.B. (Ed.). Special problems in rehabilitation. Springfield, Ill.: Charles C Thomas, 1974.

7. Derrick, W.S. Relief of pain. The Cancer Bulletin, 1974, 26, 119-120.

8. Dorland's illustrated medical dictionary (24th ed.). Philadelphia and London: W.B. Saunders Co., 1966.

9. Fischer, H.K. The problem of pain from the psychiatrist's viewpoint. Psychosomatics, 1968, 9, 319-325.

10. Grzesiak, R.C. The psychology of pain. In A.B. Cobb (Ed.), Special problems in rehabilitation. Springfield, Ill.: Charles C Thomas, 1974.

11. Hall, T.C. Philosophy of pain control in cancer patients. Postgraduate Medicine, 1970, 48 (5), 223-227.

12. Melzack, R. The perception of pain. Scientific American, 1961, 204 (2) 41-49.

13. Rusk, H.A. Rehabilitation and convalescence: the third phase of medical care. In A. Weider (Ed.), Contributions toward medical psychology (Vol 1). New York: Ronald Press, 1953.

14. Szasz, T.S. Pain and pleasure. New York: Basic Books, 1957.

Suggested Readings

Krupp, N.E. Psychiatric implications of chronic and crippling illness. Psychosomatics, 1968, 9, 109-113.

Sacerdote, P. Theory and practice of pain control in malignancy and other protracted or recurring painful illnesses. International Journal of Clinical and Experimental Hypnosis, 1970, 18, 160-180.

Woody, R.H. Psychobehavioral counseling and therapy. New York: Appleton-Century-Crofts, 1971.

Chapter 6

DEATH AND DYING

Introduction

The dying person is a living person, having a past and present history, talents and idiosyncracies, interests, and viewpoints. The dying person is a human being who has rights and opinions, who needs to be loved, talked to and cared for, and who needs acceptance. The dying person is also unique: "To be a therapist to a dying patient makes us aware of the uniqueness of each individual in this vast sea of humanity."[9(pp246-247)]

It is impossible to reconcile the differing viewpoints of persons who are identified with the slogan "death with dignity" and those who contend that there is no death with dignity.[5] The modern philosophy is that the physician should accept death as a natural and inevitable phenomenon. Even so, he must continue to strive for the preservation of life and for the increased knowledge that will make such a goal possible.[7] At the same time, it is the patient's well-being that is of first importance. His position must be evaluated from medical, psychological, social, and economic standpoints.

This chapter is not intended to present supporting evidence for either viewpoint. The reader is cautioned, however, that current treatments, designed to prolong the patient's life beyond normal limits, may be inconsistent with the physician's personal attitudes towards death with dignity. Every effort must be exerted to prevent the patient from becoming involved in the dilemma of death with dignity and natural, possibly painful death.

Patients and families are aware when life is waning and death is approaching. Death may follow a prolonged illness, or it may come very sud-

denly. When death occurs, the survivors experience shock and disbelief--
just as they did when cancer was first diagnosed. The actual fact of death
is usually more than the mind can immediately accept.

The act of death and the act of dying should not be confused. Although
death itself is singular and final, team members can help the patient through
the act of dying. Team members should not feel that their efforts have
been in vain when a patient dies, but should remember the positive contact
they have had with the patient. The importance of helping the patient
through the act of dying so that he may live fully the days before his death
and then may die peacefully should be realized by everyone involved.[4]
Good two-way communication among all persons facilitates this type of help.

Communication

Both verbal and nonverbal communication become extremely important in
the life of a dying person. When there are open channels of communication,
the terminal patient is better able to tolerate the fact that he is incurable. For many patients, the real inner self becomes revealed only as the
patient is dying.[4] The patient's whole life may pass in review before his
eyes, and he may see himself objectively for the first time.

The majority of initial communications with the patient may be based
on simply getting to know him better. Patients usually give some clues
regarding what to talk about.[11] However, most dying persons who bring up
the issues of death want to talk about them.[6]

The fears common to dying persons have been presented in Chapter 2,
"Understanding the Patient with Cancer." Highest ranked fears were:
(1) being left alone to die, (2) pain, and (3) suffocation.[6] In general,
dying becomes a lonely and impersonal experience because the patient is

often taken out of his familiar environment and put in the sterile atmosphere of the hospital,[9] where not enough emphasis is placed on the patient's needs, reactions, and experiences. For most persons, dying is perceived as an isolated and lonely experience.[11]

The problem of death is currently receiving increased interest among medical researchers. The concept of death and dying as an intrinsic part of life is emphasized in the literature and is illustrated by a more open approach within most hospital settings. The merits of this new emphasis have not been assessed. Team and family members are becoming increasingly sensitized, or willing to talk about death. They should take time to discuss death with the terminally ill patient, but only when the patient feels like talking.[9]

The supportive team members, who may be professional or family, may hesitate to talk to the patient because they don't know what to say. The following comforting guidelines may be helpful:

1. The supporting person not only should listen to what is said, but also should be alert to feelings which the patient may express by only a tone of voice, a sad look, or a tear.

2. The listener may provide information to reassure the patient regarding his treatment, prognosis, return home, etc.

3. The supporting person can "stand by" physically and emotionally and be prepared to assist the patient in any meaningful way possible.

Traditionally, the clergyman has been the prime resource for the patient and his family. His position is a difficult one because of its paradoxical nature: he seeks to represent the divine while being human; he attempts to develop insights into mysteries that are ultimately as mysterious to him as to others.   The pastor must make a concerted effort to[3]:

1. move beyond the act of ordination which sets him apart from other
    persons.

2. use meaningful communications (which may or may not be prayers)
    to relieve patients' anxieties and concerns.

3. convey to the patient that he understands his needs and values
    him as a human being.

Reinforcement and Review

6.1 What do you feel are the most important aspects to be considered when a person is dying?

    1. _____

    2. _____

6.2 Accepting the patient as a person and helping him to live fully the days before his death are greatly facilitated by:

_____ communication.

6.3 What should you do if you are hesitant about what to say to a dying patient?

_____

_____

6.4 The fears common to dying patients are:

    1. _____

    2. _____

    3. _____

6.5 The experience of dying is:

_____ and _____

6.6 Conclusions team members have currently reached regarding discussing death with the terminally ill patient are:

    1. _____

    2. _____

6.7 Guidelines to be used in communicating with the cancer patient are:

    1. _____

    2. _____

    3. _____

Answers to Questions 6.1 - 6.7

6.1 (1) accepting him as a person and (2) helping him to live fully the days before his death.

6.2 good two-way communication or open channels of communication.

6.3 Talk with him just as you would with any other patient; get to know him better.

6.4 (1) being left alone to die, (2) pain, and (3) suffocation.

6.5 lonely and isolated (or similar descriptive words conveying aloneness and impersonality).

6.6 (1) Be prepared to talk about death. (2) Talk about death only when the patient feels like talking and initiates the topic.

6.7 (1) Listen to verbal, but look for nonverbal forms of communication. (2) Be able to reassure the patient. (3) "Stand by" physically and emotionally.

Living with Death

The material presented in the following pages is general and may be applied in some manner to persons of all ages, including children. Again, the methods of understanding the patient which were presented in Chapter 2 and of communicating with the patient which were presented in Chapter 3 apply equally to the child. Even though cancer is the most frequent cause of childhood death from disease, second only to poisonings and accidents,[15] the child with a terminal disease is seldom given the same amount of time as an adult to discuss death. It is important to realize that children know when they are dying. Failure to admit to a child that he is dying will cause him to lose faith in you.

Parents of a child with catastrophic disease experience extreme emotional stress throughout the course of the child's illness. Most parents have little direct experience with death and rely heavily on team members for support. Illness disrupts family and school routines and often causes the temporary or permanent breakdown of previously harmonious relationships between family members, particularly between the parents. Crisis situations may either weaken or cement the bonds of a failing or unsuccessful marriage. The confidence of the parents and the patient in the physician is a valuable therapeutic tool that should be used to strengthen family relationships and to help family members during stressful periods.[14]

Stages of Death

The six stages of death as outlined by Kubler-Ross[9] are summarized below. The sequence represented here is not necessarily the usual one, nor is a patient in only one stage at any given point.

1. denial and isolation--Although the terminally ill patient usually

knows he is dying, he may deny the fact.[11] However, patients seldom maintain denial until the very end.[10]

2. anger--may be displaced in all directions and projected onto persons
    at random. Prolonged anger and hostile behavior may build up in
    the chronically ill patient because:

    a. The patient may feel that it is inappropriate to direct the
        anger at team members and consequently will direct the anger
        inward.

    b. Team and family members may feel that there is no acceptable
        way of allowing the patient to dispel his anger.

    c. Team members may feel that the anger is directed at them per-
        sonally, not at what they represent--health, vigor, activity,
        etc.

3. bargaining--The patient may set goals for himself and try to meet
    these goals despite physical deterioration. Goal-setting serves
    as a form of motivation. A typical example is a woman who mobi-
    lized all her energy and will power so that she could leave the
    hospital to see her son married. When she came back to the hospital
    she commented to a nurse, "I still have another son." The obvious
    implication was that she would either recover or be well enough to
    leave the hospital again to see her second son married.

4. depression--The patient shows signs of depression when he knows
    that he is becoming physically weaker and when his angry and hostile
    responses are no longer appropriate. The depression is caused by
    illness, physical separation from his family, and financial problems
    that result from dwindling financial resources and loss of job.

5. acceptance--If a patient has been given some help in working through
    the four previous stages and has had sufficient time to consider
    his status, he will reach a stage during which he is neither de-
    pressed nor angry about his "fate." His acceptance should not be
    mistaken for resignation nor for happiness, as the patient is
    almost void of feelings. He may perceive that the pain is gone,
    the struggle is over, and that it is time for "the final rest
    before the long journey."[2] He will be neither happy nor sad and
    may have little physical discomfort. If the patient can prepare
    himself slowly and is allowed to cry and grieve, then he may be
    able to decathect or separate himself from what is going on around
    him. Usually, the patient's circle of interests diminishes, and
    he prefers to be left alone and not stirred up by the problems of
    the world. He may have the courage to ask that no more relatives
    come, but perhaps only one loved one who can sit silently and com-
    fortably by his side, not speaking much, but just being there to
    look at him, smile, and touch him. Communication may become
    increasingly nonverbal. The few patients who fight until the end,
    struggle, and keep up hope seldom reach this stage of acceptance.

6. hope--Each patient should be given a chance for the most effective
    treatment possible, and hope should be maintained regardless of
    whether the patient is considered terminal or not. A patient can
    tolerate knowing he is incurable, but he can not tolerate hope-
    lessness. The nature and quality of hope are influenced by:

    a. the patient's attitude toward cancer--for example, the feeling
        that not all cancers are alike and that many patients have

lived for long periods with their disease.

b. physical factors associated with the disease and with methods
    available for treatment.

c. general attitude toward life and the will to live, which may
    be heightened by counseling and/or discussion with perceptive
    ministers or other trained persons. Patients readily sense
    indifference and rejection. The nurse, clergyman, psycholo-
    gist, psychiatrist, social worker, and rehabilitation counselor
    can be of great assistance in this area.

d. attitude and personality of the physician. Team members and
    patients who have difficulty accepting themselves as they
    really are may experience emotional problems during stressful
    periods. If the physician would accept himself as he is rather
    than as he would like to be, he would be less disturbed by
    his failures and frustrations.[13]

As mentioned previously, team members should not feel their efforts
have been in vain if the patient dies. The feeling that they did whatever
was possible whenever possible should be sufficient to dispel the feelings
of inadequacy, hopelessness, and helplessness.

Reinforcement and Review

6.8 Since one of the most common reactions to death is _____, it is logical that defense mechanisms play a major role in the patient's ultimate acceptance of death.

6.9 Why do anger and hostile behavior build up in chronically ill patients?

1. _____

2. _____

3. _____

6.10 The most common form of bargaining is:

_____.

6.11 What are the major causes of depression?

1. _____

2. _____

6.12 What does the patient's acceptance of death imply? Circle the correct response(s).

1. that he has given up
2. that he is almost void of feelings
3. that his is neither happy nor sad
4. that he is in constant pain
5. that his is neither depressed nor angry
6. that he seeks stimulation and attention
7. that he can separate himself from what is going on around him

6.13 The major factors influencing the quality and nature of hope are:

1. _____

2. _____

3. _____

4. _____

6.14 Is it possible to strike a balance between a completely realistic approach and an extremely optimistic, hopeful approach to the patient's prognosis?

      ___yes/___no

6.15 Do you feel that the increasing interest in and acceptability of the study of death is in any way damaging to the patient?

      ___yes/___no

6.16 List the stages of death:

    1. _____

    2. _____

    3. _____

    4. _____

    5. _____

    6. _____

Answers to Questions 6.8 - 6.16

6.8 denial.

6.9 (1) patient does not feel he can direct anger outward, so he directs it inward. (2) team and family members may feel there is no acceptable way of allowing the patient to dispel his anger. (3) team members may think the patient's hostile behavior is directed at them personally.

6.10 goal-setting.

6.11 (1) steadily deteriorating physical condition. (2) other emotional, economic, and/or family problems precipitated by the patient's illness.

6.12 2, 3, 5, and 7.

6.13 (1) patient's attitude toward cancer. (2) disease and its treatment. (3) attitude toward life and the will to live. (4) attitude and personality of the physician.

6.14 Yes. This approach should be similar to the guidelines presented in Chapter 3, Frames 3.11 to 3.14 regarding "What to Tell a Cancer Patient." The most important considerations are not to tell the patient anything that is patently untrue, or anything that you would have to go back on. Your nonverbal communication must get across the same message as your verbal one. The obvious approach is to be consistent.

6.15 Either yes or no. Since this question evoked your personal feelings and attitudes regarding the study of death, you may wish to determine how your philosophy fits in with current and proposed patient-care procedures and practices.

6.16 (1) denial and isolation. (2) anger. (3) bargaining. (4) depression. (5) acceptance. (6) hope.

Grief

Grief is an intense emotion that floods life when a person's inner security system is shattered by the diagnosis of cancer. Grief often starts at the time of diagnosis and may be manifest psychologically and physiologically. It may be interrupted at remission and restored later.[2] From a psychological standpoint, grief may be expressed by withdrawal, lack of appetite, insomnia, difficulty in concentrating,[2] and other reactions characterized by sorrow, fear, anxiety, guilt, and uncertainty about the future.[6] Grief may bring about physiological changes in the muscular, glandular, and cardiovascular systems.[6]

Grief is the other side of the coin of love. If you are capable of love, you are capable of grief. Profound grief is preceded by deep love which gives life meaning.[2] Grief is resolved in many different ways.

Talking about grief and death is difficult only the first time and becomes simpler with experience. Speech reduces guilt because it provides an opportunity to explain, to forgive, and be forgiven.[2] Some considerations regarding the handling of grief and related emotions are:

1. No meaningful help or assistance can be given the terminally ill patient unless his family is included. The family plays a significant role during the time of illness, and their reactions will greatly contribute to the patient's response to his illness.[9] Patients who do not have any family members on whom to rely or whose family can not or do not wish to help pose a major problem. Such patients will need additional help and understanding from team members.

2. Team and family members should be sensitive enough to recognize the

patient's verbal and nonverbal expressions of grief. They should
listen for verbal cues from the patient which will enable them to
determine the patient's willingness to face reality.

3. Family members, by talking with the team, can learn the status
    of the patient and also how they can be most effective.

4. Family members should be encouraged to express genuine emotions
    and discouraged from putting on a make-believe mask that the patient
    can see through. Through the sharing of emotions, the patient and
    his family will gradually face the reality of impending separation
    and come to an acceptance of it together.[9]

5. The patient should be supported so that he, his family, and the
    team members can work toward a dignified resolution to the problem
    of dying. The patient's efforts to stay in control as much as he
    can should be encouraged.[9]

6. Team members must provide continual reassurance and understanding
    and make life as pleasant as possible for the patient. They must
    convey to the patient that under no circumstance will he be dropped
    from treatment.[9]

7. Team and family members must not expect patients who are absorbed
    in their grief to move forward and must not blame them when they
    cannot learn. Both team members and patients must realize that
    grief increases difficulty in communication, understanding, and
    responding. It may, for example, be necessary for a physical
    therapist to repeat simple directions several times before the
    patient understands and participates in the treatment process.[2]

8. The same protections used against X-rays--time, shielding, and

distance--will soften the blow of cancer and help reduce grief.[1]
Time is required for the patient to understand and contemplate
the diagnosis of cancer; shielding is the manner in which the doctor gives the patient his diagnosis. The truth can be so gentle
that the patient's perception is that he has an enormously inter-
esting illness, one of terrific challenge to him and his doctor,
who is neither dismayed nor defeated. The truth can also be curt
and cruel. Team members can reinforce words of a thoughtful
doctor. When family members learn of the diagnosis of cancer, they
need privacy and should be some distance from the ward or clinic.
Proximity to what may be considered an unpleasant or trauma producing setting may temporarily overcome the immediate family members.

9. Prolonged and unresolved grief may be the prelude to a psychotic
break.[2] When team members recognize prolonged grief, they should
see that the patient gets specialized attention.

10. After the death of the patient, the family and friends will undoubtedly experience grief. The chaplain who ministered to the needs of
the patient should meet with the family after the death of their
loved one. His empathy and support and his suggestions for the
satisfactory resolution of grief will be of great value to the
patient's family. In addition, he may provide assistance with the
funeral arrangements and "stand by" the family for a certain period
of time.

11. Whenever possible, the family should have a period of time that
they can spend in privacy with the body before it is removed. The
feeling of shock and disbelief seldom wears off until the final

rites have been performed.[12]

Persons may need assistance in getting through the days immediately following the death of the loved one. The help may consist of words of sympathy and understanding, counseling, or assistance with rites and activities related to the funeral. Although family members rarely request sedatives or tranquilizers, the physician may wish to prescribe them.[12]

The purposes served by rituals and ceremonies (funeral) commemorating the death are: (1) the disposal of the body, (2) aid to the bereaved in reorienting themselves from the shock of the death, and (3) public acknowledgement of the death.[12]

Adjustment to the death of a loved one takes time. Some persons may adjust rapidly, some may adjust within a year or more, and some may never adjust. The specific intensity and duration of the psychological reactions experienced by the family will depend on their respective adjustment mechanisms, availability of help during the time of bereavement, and on many other personal, social, and ethnic factors.

Team members may be particularly skilled in working with the grieving family. Their skill may either be the result of professional training and/or experience. Typical ways in which the magnitude of grief may be reduced are:

1. Help the family mobilize the courage to endure the pain of having lost a loved one. Assist them in facing the full reality of what has happened.[6]

2. Help them gently break some of the bonds that tied them to the patient.[6]

3. Develop ways that will make it possible for the surviving person to find new interests, satisfactions, and creative activities until he has "bridged the gap."[6]

4. If possible, spend time with the survivors after a lapse of weeks or months to see that they have made a healthy readjustment.[8] Spending time with the survivors may not be possible, particularly if they live some distance away. However, this does not preclude communication by mail. A letter, short note, or even a post card conveying your interest would be greatly appreciated.

Wise management of grief is extremely difficult and requires infinite skill and understanding. Words of sympathy are not as important as manners, voice, and expression. Manners or personality qualities that dying persons find most helpful are[6]:

1. someone who takes an interest and has compassion.

2. someone who listens and makes an effort to get to know the patient.

3. someone who cares.

While many people have the skills and potentials listed above, few actually have or take the time to listen to what the dying person is saying. The single most important factor in the handling of grief is the attitude of "caring" and understanding which must be conveyed to the patient.

Reinforcement and Review

6.17 Think about the times you have experienced grief. How did you express it?

_____

_____

6.18 When does grief start for the cancer patient?

_____

6.19 In what basic ways may grief be expressed? Give two examples for each means of expression.

1. _____

2. _____

6.20 Is everyone capable of grief?

___yes/___no

6.21 After studying the 11 considerations pertaining to the handling of grief and related emotions, list two broad, general areas which cover the majority of these considerations. These areas may overlap slightly but can be subdivided.

1. _____

_____

2. _____

_____

6.22 List 6 of the most important considerations relating to the effective handling of grief.

1. _____

2. _____

3. _____

4. _____

5. _____

6. _____

6.23 Typical ways in which the magnitude of grief may be reduced are:

1. _____

2. _____

3. _____

4. _____

6.24 What basic personality traits and learned and/or acquired skills appear to be most helpful in the wise management of grief?

1. _____

2. _____

3. _____

Answers to Questions 6.17 - 6.24

6.17 No answer. Your own comments are sufficiently meaningful.

6.18 Grief usually starts at the time of diagnosis, but it may start later.

6.19 (1) physiologically--by changes in the muscular, glandular, and cardio-vascular systems. (2) psychologically--by withdrawal, lack of appetite, insomnia, difficulty in concentrating, and other similar symptoms.

6.20 Yes. If you are capable of love, you are capable of grief.

6.21 (1) importance of working with and enlisting the family's support (items 1, 2, 3, 4, and 5). (2) continual support and understanding and physical and psychological care from appropriate team members (items 6, 7, 8, 9, 10, and 11).

6.22 Any of the 11 are appropriate. You will obviously have included equally effective methods not provided in the presentation.

6.23 (1) help the family face the reality of the situation. (2) help them break the bonds that tied them to the patient. (3) help the surivors find new interests. (4) spend time with the survivors to make sure they have made a healthy readjustment.

6.24 (1) empathy and compassion. (2) being a good listener. (3) a "caring" attitude.

References

1. Barckley, V. Enough time for good nursing. Nursing Outlook, 1964, 12 (4), 44-48.

2. Barckley, V. Grief, a part of living. Ohio's health, 1968, 20, 34-38.

3. Byrd, J.L. Ministry to the dying patient through availability. The Cancer Bulletin, 1974, 26, 115-118.

4. Fox, J.E. Reflections on cancer nursing. Am. J. Nursing, 1966, 66, 1317-1319.

5. Freireich, Emil J Death with dignity? The Cancer Bulletin, 1974, 26 110-114.

6. Grollman, E.A. (Ed.). Concerning death: a practical guide for the living. Boston: Beacon Press, 1974.

7. Holleb, A.J. The American Cancer Society--a voluntary health agency's contribution to rehabilitation. In Rehabilitation of the cancer patient (a collection of papers presented at the Fifteenth Annual Clinical Conference on cancer). Chicago: Year Book Medical Publishers, 1972.

8. Krant, M.J. A death in the family. J.A.M.A., 1975, 231 (2), 195-196.

9. Kubler-Ross, E. On death and dying. New York: Macmillan; London: Collier Macmillan, 1969.

10. Kubler-Ross, E. What is it like to be dying? Am. J. Nursing, 1971, 71 (1), 54-60.

11. Payne, E.C., & Krant, M.J. The psychosocial aspects of advanced cancer. J.A.M.A., 1969, 210 (7), 1238-1242.

12. Schmale, A.H. Coping reactions of the cancer patient and his family. In Catastrophic illness in the seventies; critical issues and complex decisions; proceedings of the fourth national symposium. New York: Cancer Care, Inc., 1971.

13. Stehlin, J.S., & Beach, K.H. Psychological aspects of cancer therapy. J.A.M.A., 1966, 197, 100.

14. Taylor, G.H. The mother and father of a child with catastrophic disease. The Cancer Bulletin, 1974, 26, 107-109.

15. van Eys, J. The dying child. The Cancer Bulletin, 1974, 26, 105-106.

Suggested Readings

Ablin, A.R., Binger, C.M., Stein, R.C., Kushner, J.H., Zoger, S., & Mikkelson, C. A conference with the family of a leukemic child. Am. J. Dis. Child., 1971, 122, 362-364.

Barckley, V. What can I say to the cancer patient? Nursing Outlook, 1958, 6, 316-318.

Binger, C.M., Ablin, A.R., Feuerstein, R.C., Kushner, J.H., Zoger, S., & Mikkelson, C. Childhood leukemia: emotional impact on patient and family. New Eng. J. of Med., 1969, 280 (8), 414-418.

Cutter, F. Coming to terms with death: how to face the inevitable with wisdom and dignity. Chicago: Nelson-Hall, Inc., 1974.

Hendin, D. Death as a fact of life. New York: Warner Paperback Library, 1974.

Holleb, A.I. Editorial. Ca--A Cancer Journal for Clinicians, 1974, 24 (4), 256.

Marshall, H.R. Family practice and problems of aging. Postgraduate Medicine, 1975, 57 (4), 144, 147-149.

Marshall, J.R. The geriatric patient's fears about death. Postgraduate Medicine, 1975, 57 (5), 144-149.

Troup, Stanley B., & Greene, W.A. (Eds.). The patient, death, and the family. New York: Scribner's, 1974.

CHAPTER TESTS

Test questions have been developed for each chapter. The following standard instructions are to be used for each chapter test.

READ EACH OF THE FOLLOWING QUESTIONS. SELECT THE BEST ANSWER AND RECORD IT IN THE APPROPRIATE SPACE ON THE ANSWER SHEET. THERE IS ONLY ONE CORRECT ALTERNATIVE FOR EACH QUESTION.

The answer sheet on page 177 may be used for pre- and post-testing. Even numbered questions may be used for the pre-test and odd numbered questions for the post-test, or conversely. The answer sheet has been printed on both sides. Answers to the questions follow the last page of the test.

Chapter 1, "What is Cancer?"

1. Cancer can be defined as:

    A. a normal growth of cellular tissue which invades vital body organs
    B. a contagious disease
    C. an abnormal growth of cellular tissue
    D. a growth of mosaic cells which metastasizes to vital body organs and causes death
    E. the study of a large variety of tumors or swellings of a malignant nature

2. Oncology is:

    A. a method used in diagnosing cancer
    B. the study of a large variety of tumors or swellings of a malignant nature with the potentiality of causing death
    C. the study of malignant and benign tumors
    D. a new method of treating cancer
    E. the study of the history of cancer

3. Cancer may be caused by:

    A. hereditary and viral factors
    B. chemical factors and repeated injury to tissue or bone
    C. chemical and radiation factors
    D. A and B
    E. A and C

4. The two main types of cancer are:

    A. carcinoma and sarcoma
    B. leukemia and metastatic
    C. adenocarcinoma and osteogenic sarcoma
    D. sarcoma and leukemia
    E. osteogenic sarcoma and carcinoma

5. The type of cancer that invades the skin and linings of hollow organs and passageways is:

    A. sarcoma
    B. osteogenic sarcoma
    C. leukemia
    D. carcinoma
    E. Hodgkin's disease

6. The type of cancer that attacks the bone, muscle, cartilage, and lymph system is:

    A. osteogenic sarcoma
    B. carcinoma
    C. leukemia
    D. Wilm's tumor
    E. sarcoma

7. Cancer is spread by:

    A. metastasis
    B. infiltration
    C. viruses
    D. A and B
    E. A and C

8. The main purpose of an histological diagnosis is to:

    A. use it as a basis for planning surgery
    B. determine the type and extent of cancer
    C. assess only the extent of metastasis
    D. determine lymph node involvement
    E. provide information for staging

9. The most common parameter used to measure survival rate is:

    A. 1-year
    B. 2-year
    C. 5-year
    D. 7-year
    E. 10-year

10. Localized cancers are:

    A. completely curable in all instances
    B. highly curable
    C. moderately curable
    D. occasionally curable
    E. never curable

11. When cancer is in a regionalized stage, curability is:

    A. increased by 75% or more
    B. increased by 60% or more
    C. increased by 25% or more
    D. reduced by 50% or more
    E. reduced by 25% or more

12. More than half of all cancer deaths occur after the age of:

    A. 65 years of age
    B. 60 years of age
    C. 55 years of age
    D. 50 years of age
    E. 45 years of age

13. The approximate percentage of persons who contract cancer who could be saved with early diagnosis and prompt treatment is:

    A. 70%
    B. 50%
    C. 25%
    D. 15%
    E. 10%

14. Current survival rates for persons who have contracted cancer are:

    A. 4 in 5
    B. 3 in 4
    C. 2 in 3
    D. 1 in 2
    E. 1 in 3

15. In America, the number one and number two causes of death are (respectively):

    A. accidents and cancer
    B. respiratory diseases and accidents
    C. heart disease and cancer
    D. vascular lesions affecting the central nervous system and cancer
    E. cancer and influenza and pneumonia

16. Excluding superficial skin cancer and carcinoma-in-situ of the uterine cervix, the approximate number of cases of cancer in 1975 will be:

    A. 1,000,000
    B.   850,000
    C.   650,000
    D.   500,000
    E.   300,000

17. Approximately what percentage of deaths in America are caused by cancer?

    A. 25%
    B. 10%
    C. 6%
    D. 17%
    E. 33%

18. How many Americans are currently under medical care for cancer?

    A.   500,000
    B.   750,000
    C. 1,000,000
    D. 1,500,000
    E. 2,000,000

19. How many Americans are presently without evidence of cancer five years following diagnosis and treatment?

    A. 1,000,000
    B. 1,500,000
    C. 2,000,000
    D. 2,500,000
    E. 3,000,000

20. For men, the most common major site of cancer is:

    A. colon and rectum
    B. prostate
    C. digestive tract
    D. skin
    E. lung

21. For women, the most common major site of cancer is:

    A. uterus
    B. breast
    C. colon and rectum
    D. urinary
    E. lung

22. Since 1930, the age-adjusted rates for men reveal_____, which is primarily attributable to cancer of the _____.

    A. 60% increase, lung
    B. 40% increase, lung
    C. 20% increase, colon and rectum
    D. 20% increase, prostate
    E. 10% decrease, leukemia

23. Since 1936, the age-adjusted cancer rates for women reveal a _____,
    which is primarily attributable to detection of cancer of the _____.

    A. 30% decrease, breast
    B. 20% decrease, breast
    C. 30% decrease, cervix
    D. 15% decrease, cervix
    E. 10% decrease, uterus

24. Common methods of treating cancer are:

    A. surgery
    B. radiation therapy
    C. chemotherapy
    D. immunotherapy
    E. all of these

25. The quality of survival includes:

    A. general status of the patient for the first year only
    B. status of the patient 5 to 10 years following treatment
    C. only his immediate concerns such as health and comfort
    D. meaningful employment or rewarding use of time
    E. B and D

26. A Cancer Control Program, was developed within the National Cancer
    Institute for the purpose of:

    A. research and dissemination of research findings
    B. determining the cause of cancer
    C. therapy in the area of rehabilitation medicine
    D. diagnosis and treatment
    E. cooperating with health agencies in the diagnosis, prevention and
       treatment of cancer

27. The American Cancer Society is:

    A. not a research organization
    B. dedicated only to determining the cause of cancer
    C. a volunteer health organization dedicated to the control and
       eradication of cancer
    D. devoted only to finding more effective ways to treat cancer
    E. none of these

28. Earliest written records containing descriptions of cancer:

    A. date back to the Middle Ages
    B. were Percivall Patt's discovery of scratal cancer in chimney sweeps
    C. may be traced to Hippocrates
    D. date back to 2500 B.C.
    E. were found in Galen's written documents

Chapter 2, "Understanding The Patient With Cancer"

29. The diagnosis of cancer is often associated with:

    A. decreased physical ability
    B. impairment of mental functions
    C. death and dying
    D. loss of self-esteem
    E. A and B

30. Because of the potential for debilitation and uncertainty of outcome, cancer patient's problems are usually considered to exceed those of other patients in terms of:

    A. intensity
    B. frequency
    C. duration
    D. all of the above
    E. none of the above

31. Which of the following needs identified by Maslow is interpreted by the cancer patient as being most meaningful?

    A. physiological and safety
    B. safety and security
    C. security and belongingness
    D. belongingness and physiological
    E. self-actualization and security

32. Which of the following statements is true?

    A. few patients want to know if they have cancer
    B. nearly all patients with malignant disease have some knowledge of it
    C. all patients know a great deal about the treatment process
    D. most patients interpret their diagnosis of cancer in the same way
    E. most patients are not interested in the treatment process

33. Some of the most frequently occurring perceptions reported by cancer patients are those which relate to:

    A. rejection and isolation
    B. acceptance
    C. extreme pain
    D. understanding
    E. hostility

34. The most frequently occurring reaction(s) experienced by patients after learning that they have cancer are:

    A. feelings of hopelessness
    B. feelings of being "stunned," "dizzy," or "numb all over"
    C. feelings of guilt
    D. feeling of fear, anxiety, and uncertainty
    E. all of the above

35. The ego-defensive mechanisms most commonly used by cancer patients are:

    A. projection, intellectualization, and dissociation
    B. sublimation, rejection, and projection
    C. denial, sublimation, and rationalization
    D. denial, repression, and avoidance
    E. intellectualization, rationalization, and rejection

36. What factor best characterizes a satisfactory adjustment to the diagnosis of cancer?

    A. a complete lack of concern about the nature of the disease
    B. an intelligent approach in which anxiety is controlled
    C. submissive behavior characterized by a steadily decreasing frequency of emotional outbursts
    D. complete cooperation with team members
    E. acceptance of the disease and return to regressive behavior

37. The major factors to be considered in the patient's adjustment to the diagnosis of cancer are:

    A. vocational, religious, and aesthetic
    B. social, aesthetic, and physical strength
    C. personal (physical and psychological), vocational, and social
    D. physical strength, vocational, and social
    E. mental alertness, social, and aesthetic

38. Within the hospital or clinic setting, the most important effective factor in the care of a cancer patient is his relationship with his:

    A. nurse
    B. physical therapist
    C. physician
    D. psychologist
    E. radiation therapist

39. The person with whom the patient has the most frequent contact is:

    A. physician
    B. nurse
    C. social worker
    D. occupational therapist
    E. chaplain

40. The major considerations in establishing behavioral objectives are:

   A. the identification and description of observable performance
   B. your descriptions and the patient's descriptions of performance
   C. the extent to which the performance meets expectations and the
      frequency a certain behavior occurs
   D. the identification and description of observable actions and
      determination of the level of acceptable performance
   E. the identification of subjective and objective behaviors

41. Within the hospital environment, the most appropriate definition of
   motivation would be based on:

   A. drive reduction
   B. competence, or the patient's capacity to interact effectively with
      his environment
   C. psychoanalysis
   D. behaviorism
   E. Maslow's hierarchy of needs

42. In general, attitudes are:

   A. relatively resistant to change
   B. easily changed, particularly when the patient realizes it is
      necessary to adopt a new method of responding
   C. totally inflexible
   D. easy to change, as it is relatively simple to change the patient's
      physical environment and then produce the desired change
   E. relatively easy to change, as authority figures play a major role
      in facilitating attitude change

43. Attempts at attitude change will not be successful unless:

   A. authority figures are always available to induce change
   B. the patient has received appropriate counseling and psychotherapy
      prior to the introduction of change
   C. the patient understands why it is important to change his behavior
   D. all family members support the proposed change
   E. the change brings about improved levels of mental and physical
      functioning

44. Change cannot be effective unless:

   A. changed behavior is reinforced
   B. the environment is conductive or supportive to changed behavior
   C. patients are encouraged to be physically and mentally active
   D. patients are discouraged from being preoccupied with their own
      problems
   E. all of the above

Chapter 3, "Communication"

45. A vital component in the communication process is:

    A. frequency
    B. duration
    C. intensity
    D. feedback
    E. distortion

46. The three major links in the communication process are:

    A. sender, receiver, and distortion
    B. sender, receiver, and channel
    C. feedback, channel, and sender
    D. sender, receiver, and noise
    E. none of the above

47. The most common barrier(s) to effective communication with cancer patients:

    A. physical, as the sender is physically prevented from communicating with the potential receiver
    B. semantics, as persons interpret words differently
    C. emotional, because of defenses such as denial, avoidance, and repression
    D. the hospital setting--inability to talk with team members and the patient's failure to listen to what is being communicated
    E. negative attitudes and hearing loss

48. Possible barriers to effective communication which may be overcome with effort and understanding by the speaker and the listener:

    A. age differences
    B. dissonance in socio-cultural values
    C. semantics
    D. ethnic differences
    E. all of these

49. Information conveyed in a communication will more likely be accepted by the listener:

    A. when the listener can hear you
    B. when the sender or speaker is from your same socio-cultural background
    C. when the atmosphere is conductive to communication
    D. when the information is given by an authority figure such as a physician, nurse, parent, spouse, etc.
    E. when there are no problems with semantics

50. One of the most important guidelines regarding disclosure of the diagnosis to the patient is:

   A. that he may be told when you think he will be a receptive listener
   B. that the best time to tell him is when his family is around
   C. that he should not be told anything until an histological diagnosis has been established
   D. that you should always answer any questions the patient asks directly and honestly rather than referring him to a team member who may be more skilled in responding to his questions, and in discussing his diagnosis
   E. that if his condition is hopeless, he should be told as it is wrong to build up false hope

51. Based on surveys, approximately what percentage of patients want to know their diagnoses:

   A.   5% - 10%
   B. 20% - 30%
   C. 45% - 50%
   D. 60% - 75%
   E. 85% - 90%

52. Physicians' practices of revealing the diagnosis to the cancer patient are:

   A. quite standard, as there are National Cancer Institute guidelines in this area
   B. very similar within institutions, particularly within large cancer centers
   C. somewhat variable, as each physician uses his preferred plan and has his own views on the content and timing of discussions
   D. very standard, as information is always withheld when the prognosis is poor
   E. relatively standard, as when patients are terminal, they are always told immediately, and when the prognosis is good, they are always given 5-year survival data

53. The relationship between incidence of severe emotional problems, or possible suicide and being told the diagnosis is:

   A. high, with the correlation being about .80
   B. moderately high, with the correlation being about .60
   C. moderately low, with the correlation being about .30
   D. low, with the correlation being about .15
   E. negligible

54. In the initial stage of cancer, patient's communications to team and family members are:

    A. direct and truthful
    B. indirect and distorted
    C. withheld, as the patient is very depressed
    D. distorted, as communications may be distorted by the process of rationalization and regression
    E. none of these

55. In the terminal stage of cancer, patient's communications to team and family members are:

    A. direct, truthful, and not distorted because the patient knows he is going to die
    B. minimal, as the patient is frequently silent and uncommunicative
    C. always two-way, as the patient wishes to communicate with team members since he feels isolated and rejected
    D. never based on denial, as the patient wishes to talk about death
    E. relatively free and open, as the patient always accepts the reality of death without any appearance of anxiety

56. The chronically ill patient frequently exhibits:

    A. submissive behavior as most patients are extremely depressed at all times
    B. hyperactive behavior and frequently are prescribed tranquilizers
    C. paranoid behavior
    D. prolonged anger and hostile behavior
    E. manic depressive behavior

57. Manifestations of grief are evidenced by physiological changes in the:

    A. muscular, glandular and cardiovascular systems
    B. G.I. tract, endocrine system and sensory receptors
    C. muscular, cardiovascular and digestive systems
    D. endocrine, digestive and cardiovascular systems
    E. none of these

58. Communication with the cancer patient:

    A. is only verbal
    B. is only nonverbal
    C. may be both verbal and nonverbal
    D. is half verbal and half nonverbal
    E. is more nonverbal than verbal

59. General findings on verbal communication with the cancer patient are:

    A. most dying persons who bring up the issues of death want to talk
       about them
    B. team members can help the patient by letting him talk about cancer
       and death when he is ready to do so
    C. patients should not be ignored when expressing feelings about death
    D. A and B
    E. A, B, and C

60. One of the most important forms of communicating with the dying person
    is:

    A. eye contact
    B. gestures
    C. facial expressions
    D. shared silences
    E. touching

Chapter 4, "Personality and Adjustment"

61. Which of the following are typically included in definitions of personality:

    A. dynamic
    B. individual differenced
    C. perception and cognition
    D. uniqueness of response
    E. all of the above

62. With respect to individual differences, what characteristics distinguish
    cancer patients from other persons:

    A. hyperactivity
    B. impaired kinesthetic sense
    C. intelligence
    D. personality
    E. none of the above

63. Source traits:

    A. underlie surface traits and are not expressed directly
    B. are similar to surface traits
    C. are inferred from actual observations of behavior
    D. are dynamic
    E. encompass the concept of homeostasis

64. The best definition of self is:

    A. the image a person carries around with him of his own attributes
    B. the central nucleus around which the personality develops
    C. the conscious component of personality
    D. the unconscious component of personality
    E. the earliest form of body image

65. The best definition of conscious self-image is:

    A. opposite to the unconscious self-image
    B. the central nucleus around which the personality develops
    C. the image a person carries around with him of his own attributes
    D. the earliest form of body image
    E. the conscious component of personality

66. Negative self-images develop when:

    A. persons do not get along well with others
    B. not all behavior is positively reinforced
    C. when behavior is negatively reinforced
    D. patient's perceptions are either inaccurate and/or not correctly interpreted
    E. treatment procedures cause physical and emotional discomfort

67. Emotion may be defined as:

    A. a state of fear
    B. an acute condition characterized by total disruption of everyday experiences and activities
    C. a state of tension characterized by apprehension and fearfulness
    D. a fear which is tied to a specific stimulus
    E. an activated state underlying experiences and actions occurring in fear, rage, grief, love, etc.

68. Anxiety may be defined as:

    A. a state of emotional tension characterized by fearlessness
    B. an emotional state in which there is a vague, generalized feeling of fear
    C. an emotion that is frequently tied to a specific stimulus
    D. emotional responsiveness
    E. a psychotic and/or neurotic illness

69. The most accurate nonverbal measure of anxiety are:

    A. facial expressions and gestures
    B. body movements and steadiness
    C. palmar sweating and blood pressure
    D. voice pitch and steadiness
    E. gestures and blood pressure

70. The most effective way of decreasing anxiety is through:

    A. relaxation techniques and oral medication
    B. exercise and behavior modification
    C. electrical stimulation and exercise
    D. psychosurgery and oral medication
    E. behavior modification and psychosurgery

                    Chapter 5, "Pain"

71. The classification of pain into organic and psychogenic categories:

    A. usually results in errors in patient management
    B. greatly facilitates the development of a comprehensive operational
       definition of pain
    C. eliminates the tendency to rely on introspective reports
    D. is inconsistent with the medical model
    E. B and C

72. Pathological bone fracture, necrosis, and compression of spinal sensory
    nerve roots are examples of:

    A. psychogenic pain
    B. organic pain
    C. phantom pain
    D. psychologic pain
    E. psychodynamic pain

73. Separating physical pain from fear of pain is:

    A. very easy
    B. quite easy
    C. not very hard
    D. quite difficult
    E. very difficult

74. Quality and intensity of pain are influenced by:

    A. patient's past history
    B. meaning pain has for the patient
    C. patient's present state of mind
    D. A and B
    E. A, B, and C

75. Pain thresholds are:

    A. about the same for most persons
    B. subject to inter-individual and intra-individual differences
    C. the same for augmenters and reducers
    D. lower in well adjusted persons
    E. the same at night as they are in the daytime

76. Which of the following factors could influence pain thresholds:

    A. verbal instructions such as hypnosis
    B. biofeedback
    C. analgesics
    D. A and B
    E. A, B, and C

77. Phantom pain is considered to be:

    A. imaginary, as pain can not be experienced in a limb that has been amputated
    B. experienced only by persons who have paranoid tendencies
    C. psychogenic rather than chronic
    D. real and may be chronic
    E. more psychological than real

78. In most instances, the physical source of pain is:

    A. uncertain, as patients have difficulty describing locations of pain
    B. somewhat uncertain, as patients may not know what is causing the pain
    C. relatively easy to determine, as the patient and the physician readily understand the meaning of words used to describe pain and other symptoms
    D. obvious, such as pain resulting from surgery
    E. none of these

79. Use of narcotics in pain control:

    A. seldom causes any addiction problems
    B. sometimes causes addiction problems
    C. usually causes addiction problems
    D. always causes addiction problems
    E. is completely unpredictable, because of individual differences, drug interactions and other complex and interrelated variables

80. Techniques used by physical therapists to control pain in patients include:

    A. electrical stimulation, exercise, and hypnosis
    B. precutaneous cordotomy, postural correction, and traction
    C. applications of heat and cold, massage, and hydrotherapy
    D. acupuncture, biofeedback, and hypnosis
    E. dorsal rhizotomy, radiotherapy, and hydrotherapy

81. Chronic pain:

    A. is related to underlying somatic pathology
    B. responds to appropriate medical treatment
    C. is disproportionate to the physical illness, and does not respond to appropriate medical treatment
    D and E on the next page

D. is similar to psychological pain, as it does not respond to appropriate medical treatment
E. is not treatable, as the physician generally assumes that the pain is not real

82. Palliation may be defined as:

A. methods which provide relief from pain but do not cure
B. methods of curing rather than providing relief
C. methods of controlling pain by using only analgesics
D. methods of controlling pain by using surgery and chemotherapy
E. methods of controlling pain by using surgery, chemotherapy and radiation therapy

83. A relatively new approach in alleviating chronic, intractable pain involves:

A. a rehabilitation team which mobilizes health professionals in the psychosocial and occupational/vocational areas
B. use of psychiatrists and psychologists to determine the cause of pain
C. a multidisciplinary team composed of specialists
D. working with the family to determine the patient's history of pain, and testing out various methods of pain control on the patient
E. determining the source of the pain through introspective methods and psychological tests

Chapter 6, "Death and Dying"

84. In many instances, when the patient realizes that he is dying:

A. he discovers his inner self and may see himself objectively for the first time
B. he does not wish to communicate with anyone, and withdraws
C. his need to be accepted as a person is greatly decreased
D. he does not wish to live fully the days before his death
E. he has no major fears, and accepts death naturally

85. The majority of persons perceive death as:

A. natural, and realistically accept the fact of death
B. a lonely and isolated experience
C. unrealistic, as they know that life can always be prolonged despite cost
D. a welcome relief to the pain and suffering they have experienced
E. none of these

86. Fear(s) most commonly experienced by dying persons:

A. being left alone to die
B. extreme and prolonged pain and suffering
C, D, and E on the next page

C. disfigurement and change in body image and body function
D. helplessness
E. all of the above

87. Within the last few years, greater effort has been exerted in the study of death. Assuming that the topic of death is approached with sensitivity and caution, the most realistic outcome is that:

A. team members can initiate conversations about death at any time
B. the family can talk about death in front of the patient without upsetting him
C. the topic of death may be discussed more realistically, but all discussions should be avoided unless the patient brings up the topic and wishes to talk about death
D. team members are now capable of providing assurance to the patient at any time
E. team members are now trained to "stand by" the patient during crisis situations that may result in the patient's death

88. The most effective way to reduce the majority of severe physical discomfort associated with death is with:

A. psychotherapy
B. tranquilizers
C. good physical therapy
D. good nursing care
E. a spinal nerve block

89. The first of the six stages of death outlined by Kubler-Ross is:

A. anger
B. denial and isolation
C. bargaining
D. hope
E. acceptance

90. The last of the six stages of death outlined by Kubler-Ross:

A. denial and isolation
B. depression
C. anger
D. hope
E. bargaining

91. Most pediatric patients:

A. are generally difficult to communicate with, and do not wish to talk about death
B. should not be told they are dying
C. have families who usually have had experience in handling death, so no communication difficulties are experienced
D and E on the next page

D. like adults, do know they are dying
E. unlike adults, do not know they are dying

92. In observations of pediatric patients, one of the most valuable therapeutic tools is:

A. the confidence parents and the patient have in the physician
B. counseling and psychotherapy sessions which may be arranged with the psychologist
C. good care and lots of attention from parents and friends
D. telling the child that he has cancer and discussing death with him
E. discussing death with the child as soon as the diagnosis of cancer has been made

93. The main reason for the build-up of hostile behavior in the chronically ill patient is:

A. he is upset with himself because he has cancer
B. family members are not expert at letting him express his hostility outward
C. the patient feels that it is inappropriate to direct anger at team members, and consequently directs anger inwardly
D. the patient's behavior is slightly neurotic, and it is reasonable that he would direct hostile behavior inwardly
E. there is no possible way for him to physically direct his hostility outwardly

94. The most frequent overt expressions of grief are:

A. fear, anxiety, sorrow, and withdrawal
B. repression, projection, and sublimation
C. fear, sorrow, and denial
D. anxiety, withdrawal, and intellectualization
E. physiological changes in the muscular, glandular, and cardiovascular systems

95. The major problem in working with the dying patient is that:

A. team members have difficulty expressing themselves verbally, and verbal communication is so much more important than nonverbal communication
B. few team and family members have compassion and take an interest in the patient
C. most team members do not recognize the fact that the patient is grieving, as only physiological measures of grief obtained from the muscular, glandular, and cardiovascular systems provide reliable, meaningful data
D. few team and family members actually take the time to listen to what the patient is saying
E. so little can be done with the grieving patient that it is better to devote time and effort to patients who are not terminal

96. No meaningful help or assistance can be given the terminally ill patient unless:

   A. his physician requests that team members provide assistance
   B. his family is included
   C. he is capable of expressing his grief openly
   D. a qualified team member is always present to talk with him about his problems
   E. he always cooperates with team and family members

ANSWER SHEET

Chapter 1

1. _____
2. _____
3. _____
4. _____
5. _____
6. _____
7. _____
8. _____
9. _____
10. _____
11. _____
12. _____
13. _____
14. _____
15. _____
16. _____
17. _____
18. _____
19. _____
20. _____
21. _____
22. _____
23. _____
24. _____
25. _____
26. _____
27. _____
28. _____

Chapter 2

29. _____
30. _____
31. _____
32. _____
33. _____
34. _____
35. _____
36. _____
37. _____
38. _____
39. _____
40. _____
41. _____
42. _____
43. _____
44. _____

Chapter 3

45. _____
46. _____
47. _____
48. _____
49. _____
50. _____
51. _____
52. _____
53. _____
54. _____
55. _____
56. _____
57. _____
58. _____
59. _____
60. _____

Chapter 4

61. _____
62. _____
63. _____
64. _____
65. _____
66. _____
67. _____
68. _____
69. _____
70. _____

Chapter 5

71. _____
72. _____
73. _____
74. _____
75. _____
76. _____
77. _____
78. _____
79. _____
80. _____
81. _____
82. _____
83. _____

Chapter 6

84. _____
85. _____
86. _____
87. _____
88. _____
89. _____
90. _____
91. _____
92. _____
93. _____
94. _____
95. _____
96. _____

178

ANSWER SHEET TO CHAPTER TESTS

Chapter 1

1. C
2. B
3. E
4. A
5. D
6. E
7. D
8. B
9. C
10. B
11. D
12. A
13. B
14. E
15. C
16. C
17. D
18. C
19. B
20. E
21. B
22. B
23. D
24. E
25. E
26. E
27. C
28. D

Chapter 2

29. C
30. D
31. C
32. B
33. A
34. E
35. D
36. B
37. C
38. C
39. B
40. D
41. B
42. A
43. C
44. E

Chapter 3

45. D
46. B
47. C
48. E
49. D
50. C
51. E
52. C
53. E
54. A
55. B
56. D
57. A
58. C
59. E
60. E

Chapter 4

61. E
62. E
63. A
64. B
65. C
66. D
67. E
68. B
69. C
70. A

Chapter 5

71. A
72. B
73. E
74. E
75. B
76. E
77. D
78. D
79. A
80. C
81. C
82. A
83. C

Chapter 6

84. A
85. B
86. E
87. C
88. D
89. B
90. D
91. D
92. A
93. C
94. A
95. D
96. B

CLASSIFICATION OF ABNORMAL REACTION PATTERNS

Disorders of psychogenic origin or without clearly defined physical cause or structural change in brain

Transient Situational Personality Disorders

Acute symptom response to an overwhelming situation in basically stable personality.
Gross stress reaction—reactions to combat or to civilian catastrophes.
Adjustment reaction of infancy—undue apathy, excitability, feeding or sleeping difficulties of psychogenic origin.
Adjustment reaction of childhood—habit disturbances (nail-biting), conduct disturbances (truancy), neurotic traits (tics).
Adjustment reaction of adolescence—transient reactions due to adolescent conflicts.
Adult situational reaction—maladjustment to difficult situation.
Adjustment reaction of later life—reactions to environmental demands of later life.

Psychoneurotic Disorders (Neuroses)

Chief characteristic is anxiety, directly felt or unconsciously controlled by use of various psychological defense mechanisms. No gross disorganization of personality or loss of contact with reality.
Anxiety reaction—diffuse anxiety often punctuated by acute anxiety attacks.
Dissociative reaction—fugue, amnesia, multiple personality, somnambolism.
Conversion reaction—anxiety converted into functional symptoms of illness.
Phobic reaction—persistent fears despite individual's realization that they are irrational.
Obsessive-compulsive reaction—persistent, irrational thoughts and impulses.
Depressive reaction—extreme dejection over environmental setback or loss.
Psychoneurotic reaction, other.

Psychophysiologic Autonomic and Visceral Disorders ("Psychosomatic Disorders")

Structural change following chronic, exaggerated physiological expression of emotion; the emotion is repressed and discharged through viscera.
Skin reaction, such as atopic dermatitis.
Musculoskeletal reaction, as tension headaches.
Respiratory reaction, as hiccoughs.
Cardiovascular reaction, as hypertension.
Hemic and lymphatic reaction, as diffuse changes in blood systems.
Gastrointestinal reaction, as chronic gastritis.
Genitourinary reaction, as menstrual disturbances.
Endocrine reaction, as obesity.
Nervous system reaction, as general fatigue.
Reaction of organs of special sense, as physical changes in retinae or eardrums.

Psychotic Disorders (Functional Psychoses)

Personality disintegration with disorientation for time, place, and/or person. Hospitalization ordinarily required.
Schizophrenic reactions—a group of psychotic reactions involving withdrawal from reality, disturbances in thought processes, and emotional blunting and distortion.
  1 Simple type—apathy and indifference without conspicuous delusions or hallucinations.
  2 Hebephrenic type—severe disorganization with silliness, mannerisms, delusions, hallucinations.
  3 Catatonic type—conspicuous motor behavior with excessive motor activity and excitement or generalized inhibition and stupor.
  4 Paranoid type—poorly systematized delusions; often hostility and aggression.
  5 Acute indifferentiated type—sudden schizophrenic reaction which may clear up or develop into other definable type.
  6 Chronic undifferentiated type—chronic, mixed symptomatology not fitting other types.
  7 Schizo-affective type—admixture of schizophrenic and affective reactions.
  8 Childhood type—schizophrenic reactions occurring before puberty.

9 Residual type—mild residual symptoms following more severe cases.
Paranoid reactions—persistent delusions usually without hallucinations. Behavior and emotional responses consistent with delusions. Intelligence well preserved.
  1 Paranoia—well systematized delusions, generally of persecution or grandeur.
  2 Paranoid state—transient paranoid delusions, not well systematized, lacking the bizarre fragmentation of the schizophrenic.
Affective reactions—exaggerations of mood with related thought disturbance.
  1 Manic depressive reaction—prolonged periods of excitement or depression or mixture or alternation of the two.
  2 Psychotic depressive reaction—severe depression and delusions of unworthiness.
Involutional psychotic reaction—depression in involutional period without previous psychosis.

Personality Disorders (Character Disorders)

Developmental defects or pathological trends in the personality structure rather than decompensation under stress. Lifelong pattern of "acting out" with little or no anxiety.
Special symptom reaction—disturbances where specific symptom is the outstanding expression of pathology, like stuttering, nail-biting, enuresis, tics.
Personality pattern disturbance—personality types that can rarely be basically altered by therapy and tend to decompensate to psychosis under stress. (Inadequate personality, schizoid personality, cyclothymic personality, paranoid personality.)
Personality trait disturbance—emotional immaturity with inability to maintain emotional equilibrium and independence under even minor stress. (Emotionally unstable personality, passive-aggressive personality, compulsive personality, other personality trait disturbance.)
Sociopathic personality disturbance—inability to conform to prevailing social standards; lack of social responsibility.
  1 Antisocial reaction—impulsive, unable to profit from experience or feel real loyalty.
  2 Dyssocial reaction—criminals from abnormal environment with good ego strength.
  3 Sexual deviation—any of wide range of sexually deviant reactions.
  4 Addiction—alcoholism and drug addiction.

Disorders caused by or associated with impairment of brain tissue function

Acute Brain Disorders

Temporary, reversible, diffuse impairment of brain tissue function; orientation and intellectual functions impaired; transient delusions and hallucinations common. Acute syndromes include those associated with intracranial infection, systematic infection, drug or poison intoxication, alcohol intoxication or delirium following minimal alcohol intake without apparent pre-existing mental disorder, trauma (head injury), circulatory disturbance, convulsive disorder, metabolic disturbance, intracranial neoplasm (tumor), or unknown cause.

Chronic Brain Disorders

Result from relatively permanent, diffuse impairment of brain tissue function. Condition may become milder or more severe. Involves some degree of disturbance of memory, judgment, comprehension, and affect; neurotic, psychotic, or personality disorder reactions may be superimposed. Chronic syndromes include those associated with congenital cranial anomalies, central nervous system syphilis, other intracranial infection, intoxication by toxic agents like lead and carbon monoxide, brain trauma (head injury) with permanent damage, cerebral arteriosclerosis, other circulatory disturbance, convulsive disorder, senile brain degeneration, disturbance of metabolism or growth, or nutrition, intracranial neoplasm (tumor), or unknown cause.

Mental retardation (mental deficiency)

Involves individuals who manifest subaverage intellectual functioning which originates during the developmental period and results in impaired adaptive behavior. The APA classification of mental retardation has been superseded by the fourfold classification recommended by the President's Panel on Mental Retardation (1962): *mild* (IQ 50-70), *moderate* (IQ 35-49), *severe* (IQ 20-34), *profound* (IQ below 20).

EVALUATION OF <u>PSYCHOSOCIAL</u> <u>ASPECTS</u> <u>OF</u> <u>CANCER</u> <u>PATIENT</u> <u>CARE</u>

Read each of the following statements. Using the 7-unit scale, which ranges from 1 (low) to 7 (high), circle the number which most closely represents your evaluation of each statement.

I. CONTENT OF MATERIAL   <u>Low</u>   <u>Average</u>   <u>High</u>

		Low			Average			High
1.	comprehensiveness	1	2	3	4	5	6	7
2.	relevancy	1	2	3	4	5	6	7
3.	level of difficulty	1	2	3	4	5	6	7

Please comment on the following:

1. Is the material covered adequately? _____

_____

2. Is the material too simple or complex? _____

_____

3. Other remarks related to content: _____

_____

II. METHOD OF PRESENTATION

		Low			Average			High
1.	quality of writing	1	2	3	4	5	6	7
2.	transmission of information	1	2	3	4	5	6	7
3.	appealing to work on	1	2	3	4	5	6	7
4.	question and answer format	1	2	3	4	5	6	7

Please comment on the following:

1. Amount of material presented per page: _____

_____

2. Method of presenting questions and answers: _____

_____

3. Other remarks related to presentation: _____

_____

III. TESTING METHODS   Low   Average   High

1. coverage of information   1   2   3   4   5   6   7

2. level of difficulty   1   2   3   4   5   6   7

Please comment on the following:

1. Difficulty level of test: _____

_____

2. Content of test: _____

_____

IV. GENERAL FACTORS

1. Approximately how long did it take to work through the text? _____

2. Did you experience any problems? _____. If yes, please specify

pages and frame numbers: _____

3. Did you find the definitions at the end of the chapters useful?

Yes ( )   Relatively ( )   Not particularly ( )   No ( )

4. Do you plan to look up any of the references presented at the end

of the chapters?

Yes ( )   Probably Will ( )   Probably Will Not ( )   No ( )

5. Do you plan to do any of the suggested readings?

Yes ( )   Probably Will ( )   Probably Will Not ( )   No ( )

6. Please specifiy what you liked most about this text: _____

_____

7. Please specify what you liked least about this text: _____

_____

8. Please comment on any aspect related to the content, method of

presentation, and testing methods not previously covered by this

evaluation: _____

_____